Benzo Free

THE WORLD OF ANTI-ANXIETY DRUGS AND THE REALITY OF WITHDRAWAL

D E Foster

Denim Mountain Press

ERIE, COLORADO

www.BenzoFree.org

Printed in the United States of America
by Denim Mountain Press

First Printing, 2018

ISBN 978-1-7322786-1-5

Includes bibliographical references.

Denim Mountain Press
PO Box 25
Erie, Colorado 80516-0025

www.DenimMountainPress.com

Cover Design by Andy Meaden (meadencreative.com)

The author welcomes feedback including comments, personal accounts, additions, and corrections at www.BenzoFree.org

ev0102

Contents

To Mom and Dad,
thanks for believing in me.

Acknowledgments

No one is useless in this world who lightens the burdens of another.

— Charles Dickens

There are so many who have lightened my burdens. Please bear with me while I list a few of those who have made both my journey through withdrawal and the writing of this book possible.

There is only one place to start. When you marry your best friend, you've already done something right. Thank God I didn't mess that one up. I do not have the words to describe what Shana has meant to me these past five years, let alone the past twenty-two years of our marriage. I could relive this life a thousand times over, and I would never make a better decision than choosing her for my life partner. Thanks, Babe, you are the world to me.

Shana isn't the only one who supported me during this time. My family and extended family endured my seclusion, my moods, my complaints, and my absence. First off, thanks to my mom and dad for their love, encouragement, and enthusiasm for the past 50-some years and to my sister for putting up with a brother who can be selfish, moody, and distant at times. Thanks to my mother-in-law and father-in-law for their unending patience and to all my brothers-in-law, sisters-in-law, aunts, uncles, nieces, nephews, and cousins. I am now and will always be grateful for your love and understanding.

I also want to thank all my friends who helped me along the way. Thanks to John & Cindy, Jan & Mike, Christine & John, Chip & Erin, John & Gloria, our friend and traveling partner Jenn, my spiritual brother Matt, and the infectiously optimistic Hala. But most of all, thanks to my best buddy of over 30 years, J.B., who has been there when I needed him time and time again. He knows all my secrets, flaws, and shortcomings, and yet still answers the phone every time I call. I am blessed to call you all my friends.

Moving on to benzos, I must thank the one medical professional who helped me more than any other. Prof. Ashton, thank you. Your manual is a life saver. There's no other way to put it. Thousands of people are alive today and benzo-free thanks to you. I wish you a peaceful and happy retirement. God Bless.

Thanks to Dr. V, Denise, Liz, Jill, Christine, Celeste, Kathryn, and all the other medical professionals who put up with my aches and pains and didn't just brush me aside when they heard the words "benzo withdrawal." I am forever grateful, and I am now alive and recovering thanks to you.

Thanks to my fellow withdrawal sufferers who struggle every day and every night. You are the true motivation behind this book. Thank you for sharing your lives with me. I am a better person for it.

The cover of the book looks the way it does because of Andy Meaden. Thanks to him for the fantastic cover design and graphics. And thanks to my editor, proofreaders, and all the other people who helped make this book become a reality.

And in closing, I must thank Bear, my furry friend. He's eleven years old now and getting tired, but I'm hopeful he'll stick around for a while longer. You helped both Shana and me get through this difficult time, and you'll be in our hearts forever my friend. Thanks Buddy.

Oh, and one last thing. Thanks for reading my book, or at least the first few pages of it. I am forever humbled that anyone would voluntarily want to read the words I put to the page. Thank you for taking the time to hear what I have to say.

Peace,
D

Preface

Imagine that you had a car accident. A bad one. A really bad one. Your Prius took on a Mack truck hauling steel piping...and lost.

Blood is everywhere. Lacerations cover your arms, legs, and face. Bruises blend with burns leaving little unadulterated skin. Your muscles are twisted and torn. A severe concussion has left you in a fog, barely aware of your surroundings. Paramedics struggle to keep you conscious, but your mind slips into delirium. You're terrified. You don't know what happened, why this happened, or even who you are. You will survive, but your recovery will be grueling and painful at times and may take months, even years. You may lose your home, your job, even your family. You realize that the life you once knew is now gone and you will never be the same person again.

Now imagine that same pain, that same fear, that same suffering, but no one else can see it. There was no car accident. No paramedics are rushing to your aid. It all happened inside of you. When you seek help for your injuries, you're met with annoyance, disdain, and disbelief. You attempt to relate your suffering to your family, friends, and colleagues, but no one understands. How could they? Why would anybody believe this hodgepodge of bizarre, invisible, unrelated "symptoms" that you claim are making your life unbearable? And even if people believed you, they'd never accept the outlandish premise that the damage wasn't caused by some massive semi-tractor trailer truck, but instead by one tiny, little pill. A pill that your doctor ironically prescribed to make you feel better.

Welcome to the world of benzo withdrawal.

It's been a long five years. I've endured debilitating muscle spasms, torn muscles, restless legs, brain zaps, tinnitus, severe heart palpitations, burning skin, flushing, face spiders, memory loss, cognitive dysfunction, throat swelling, chronic insomnia, acute gastritis, abdominal distension, pelvic floor dysfunction, vertigo, uncharacteristic aggression and irritability, panic attacks, personality changes, and the most severe anxiety and depression in my life. I've scheduled over a hundred medical appointments with a parade of doctors, specialists, therapists, and counselors. I've been unable to work and put a burdensome strain on my family. I've faced a wall of disbelief and scorn from friends and doctors alike. I've had days when getting out of bed was a near impossible feat. And I've begged God, and anyone else who would listen, that it would all just end.

Even if this description sounds foreign and implausible to you, it's familiar to thousands of people around the world. People attempting to withdraw from a class of prescription drugs known as benzodiazepines and their cousins, nonbenzodiazepines (z-drugs) and thienodiazepines. You may know them better as Xanax, Ativan, Klonopin, Valium, Ambien, Lunesta, Restoril, Librium, and Sonata among others. Or perhaps by their street names like xannies, z bars, k-pin, qual, candy, zanbars, totem poles, K, sleepers, r2, BZDs, bennies, stupefy, tranx, zombie pills, roofies, goofballs, and downers.

Perhaps you picked up this book because you have personal experience with these drugs. Or maybe you have no experience with benzos, and my opening sounded like some hysterical hypochondriac's rant. Although benzo dependence may not be discussed commonly in most social circles, it exists, and it destroys lives.

> *Benzos are very easy to get on, almost impossible to get off. Benzo withdrawal is a beast — often terrifying, sometimes dangerous, and almost always drawn out over a very long period of time.* [1]

— Dr. Allen Frances, Professor Emeritus at Duke University, Chairman of the DSM-IV Committee

If you're currently dependent on benzos and this opening has added to your fears, I apologize because that was not my intent. Upon tackling the subject of benzodiazepine withdrawal for this book, I realized that I would be walking a very fine line. How do I share the difficulties that I and thousands of others face every day without terrorizing an already anxiety-prone audience? How do I raise awareness among the general public and soothe the struggling patient at the same time?

The truth is, I can't. All I can do here is be honest, share what I have learned, and tell my story.

During my five years tapering and recovering from clonazepam (Klonopin), I had thousands of questions, and I sought thousands of answers. This book is the direct result. It's a compilation of my experience with benzo withdrawal, what I learned from years of research and study, and stories that my friends shared with me along the way. While my withdrawal was the most painful and challenging period in my life — a period that continues as I write this book — it was not without its own rewards. I would never want to repeat the hell I've been through, but I now know I am a better person because of it.

If you, or someone you know, is dependent on a benzodiazepine or z-drug then let me just say this:

> *Expectations of withdrawal are often much worse than the actual experience itself.*

Yes, some people do have harrowing experiences and struggle with symptoms for years. But they're in the minority. Thousands of us have been through this and not only survived but thrived once it was over. We know many of the ups and downs, the dos and don'ts, and we're here to support those who follow. There are so many resources available to help, and this book is only one of them.

I don't believe anybody should be forced to withdraw from benzos if they don't want to. It's a personal decision between the patient and his or her doctor. I am glad I tapered off benzodiazepines, and I would do it again. It's great to be benzo-free.

INTRODUCTION

If You're Currently Taking Benzos, Please Read This First

Before we dive in too deep, I think it's essential to share six key pieces of information up front. I'll try and keep it brief.

1) Taper Slowly Under Doctor Supervision - I'll say this repeatedly throughout the book because it's that important. Almost every medical expert who has worked with long-term benzo patients will tell you the same thing. Stopping benzos cold turkey, especially without medical supervision, can be very dangerous. I understand the urgent desire to free yourself from this medication but quitting cold turkey will most likely make it worse. It can even be fatal. If you decide to withdraw, a slow taper under doctor supervision is the smartest choice you can make.

Abrupt cessation of benzodiazepines may be very dangerous.[2]

— Prof. C. Heather Ashton, *The Ashton Manual*

2) Not Everyone Will Have a Difficult Withdrawal - This is excellent news! It's estimated that about half of those who withdraw from long-term benzodiazepine use won't have to deal with the difficulties of benzodiazepine withdrawal syndrome (BWS). Many withdraw with little or no side effects or symptoms. Unfortunately, no one knows who will have trouble during withdrawal and who won't. So, it's always a good idea to taper slowly under medical supervision regardless.

3) Trigger Warning - The topic of this book is benzodiazepine withdrawal. It's an honest account of the journey so many of us have undertaken. If you're planning or currently in withdrawal, please read this book with caution and be aware of possible triggers.

4) Suicidal Ideation - It's not uncommon for people going through benzo withdrawal to have thoughts of suicide. Benzo withdrawal may seem hopeless at times, but it's not. It does get better. If you are having suicidal thoughts, please seek professional help immediately. Suicide prevention assistance organizations are listed in the "Resources" section of the appendix.

5) Follow *The Ashton Manual* - *The Ashton Manual* is widely considered the de facto standard for withdrawal from benzodiazepines, z-drugs, and other minor tranquilizers and is available online for free at www.benzo.org.uk/manual. I'll share more about Professor Ashton and her work throughout this book.

6) Not Medical Advice - This book is for informational purposes only and is not intended to provide medical advice. Please read the complete medical disclaimer in the front of this book for more details.

That's it. Now we can get back to the introduction. Any questions?

Sure, I have tons. But maybe we should start with the basics. In your own words, what's this book about?

This book is about benzos. About the drugs, the history, and the culture surrounding the drugs. It's about mental health and anxiety. It's about benzo withdrawal and the struggles, symptoms, and frustrations that I and so many others have faced. It's about life and the challenges that keep us up at night. It's about a positive, balanced approach to benzo withdrawal that led me, and others like me, to success.

But most of all, this book is about hope. I know that sounds a bit grandiose, but it's honest. I want this book to be about hope. Hope for the patient who is terrified, struggling, and at her wit's end. Hope for the spouse who doesn't know how much more support he can provide. Hope for the doctor who doesn't have the information to accurately help her patients. Hope for the protracted patient who just wants to know when this nightmare will end. And hope for our world in that we will finally take this problem seriously and get real help for those in need. But most of all, hope that one day no one will ever have to go through the excruciating journey of benzo withdrawal again.

Why did you decide to write a book?

During my journey through withdrawal, I had an endless array of questions. Thousands of them. Questions without answers. Should I withdraw or stay on my meds? How long should I taper? How long will this last? Is this pain from the benzos, or is it something else?

What about this pain? Is it something more serious? Should I go to the doctor about this issue? How about this one? Should I go to the ER? Why is my doctor clueless? Why doesn't my doctor believe me? Which medical tests make sense? Which can I afford? Can I have caffeine? Alcohol? Sugar? Gluten? If not now, when? Can I exercise? Should I exercise? If so, how much? If I push it will I pull a muscle? Now that I pulled a muscle, do I need physical therapy? Why am I not healing with physical therapy? Will I sleep tonight? How about tomorrow night? Anytime this week? Why did this happen to me? Will it get better? Will I survive? ...and above all else, when will it end?

Questions plague every one of us who experiences benzodiazepine withdrawal syndrome. Incessant, unending questions. As for me, I am also ADHD, which created a perfect blend of fear, anxiety, and a hyperactive mind. I would obsess about multiple worries simultaneously. It was a never-ending kaleidoscope of uncertainty. And it almost drove me mad. All these questions, and so few answers.

When I worked as a screenwriter, one of my favorite parts of the job was the research. I've grown to love research. So, every time I had a question about my withdrawal, I would dig around the Internet for answers. I would go to more doctors. I would spend hours on the benzo recovery boards. I was insatiable. Eventually, I had piles upon piles of research on benzos, anxiety, depression, addiction, happiness, positive psychology, mindfulness, medical science, legal issues, and much more. Anything that might remotely help my recovery. But then I looked around at all this information, and I asked myself, now what?

The answer was staring me in the face. I'm a writer, a benzo survivor, and I have all this research. Hmmm, I wonder what I should do? The final decision came down to one thing: I needed something good to come from this. I couldn't accept that my journey through benzo withdrawal was meaningless. It had to have a purpose. And so, *Benzo Free* was born. By the time I finished writing the first draft of the book, I'd spent four years and read and cataloged over one thousand separate articles, studies, websites, and books. It would be a real shame if all of that went to waste.

If I'm the only person who reads this book and finds it helpful, that's fine. Honestly. I'm still glad I wrote it. It's a cathartic process and just writing about it is helping me recover. But, if I'm lucky enough that others find this book helpful, then I can honestly say that the experience I went through had a purpose. Something good has come from it. And in the end, that's what really matters.

But what makes you qualified to write this book?

Nothing, professionally speaking. No degree in psychology. No medical experience. No counseling experience except a brief stint as a psychiatric technician right out of college (which qualifies me for absolutely nothing). No addiction experience. I've never worked in a rehab center nor have I ever been to one. I have absolutely no professional experience that would qualify me to write this book, nor do I claim to.

I'm just a guy who went through benzodiazepine withdrawal and decided to write about his experience and what he learned along the way. Perhaps what I learned can be useful to others.

One thing I hope the reader will keep in mind is that this is my experience. This book is my opinion. One of the steadfast rules in benzo withdrawal is that everyone's experience is different. Be careful of anyone who says that they have the "miracle cure" for benzo withdrawal. And that goes for me too. Please don't take any of what I say here as gospel. I can only relate what worked for me and others I've met and share it as objectively as I know how. Withdrawal experiences vary greatly. You'll find out what works for you along the way. It just takes time.

What's with all these questions in bold? Like this one?

When I decided to write this book, I looked at a variety of possible formats. What would the overall structure look like? How would I relay all the research I've accumulated? How do I share my story and experiences? I kept researching as I debated with myself on the issue. The storytelling approach of a novel was appealing, but it didn't allow me the organizational structure I was seeking. I wanted some format that provided for structured access to information and still allowed me a way to creatively tell my story when needed.

So, I imagined myself five years ago. Before I started to taper. Twelve years on clonazepam and scared shitless about what's to come. I was beyond desperate. I so badly wanted information. I had *The Ashton Manual,* which was a huge help, but I wanted so much more. I wanted someone to guide me through this. I wanted someone to tell me that I could make it. I wanted a calming voice to walk me through what I was about to experience.

So, I started to envision this book as a conversation. A conversation between the student — someone like me five years ago, dependent on benzos, not sure where to turn for help, desperately wanting answers — and the teacher — someone benzo-free, on the other side, perhaps a bit wiser after his experience. And thus, I settled on this conversational Q&A format. I hope you find it helpful.

Next question?

So, since this is your story, perhaps you should tell me about yourself.

Well, let's see. I'm 52-years-old, live in Colorado, and share my home with my totally awesome wife (no, she didn't make me say that) and my dog named Bear. I'm an average guy, although a bit more nomadic than most. Over the past 35 years I've held jobs as an IT director, database programmer, screenwriter, college instructor, web designer, movie producer, a/v specialist, drummer, psychiatric technician, community organizer, usher, shipping clerk, etcetera... and now I'm writing a book. See a pattern?

Most of my career has been split between working in film and computers. I've spent 25 years programming applications and databases for several large corporations. I've also spent 15 years writing screenplays, teaching screenwriting, and organizing film events. The computer work pays significantly better, but my real passions lie with teaching and writing. More recently, I have been unable to continue working as a database consultant due to complications from withdrawal. Therefore, I decided to spend my time writing this book. Sometimes bad things happen for a good reason.

What about your experience with benzos?

I initially wrote my detailed story with benzos right here in the introduction, but then I decided to move it to Part II of the book. It fits better there, and I didn't want to bore you by talking too much about myself in the opening. But still, I guess I should provide you a summary of my experience with benzos here as a reference. Check out chapter 10 for the full story.

I was prescribed clonazepam (Klonopin) for chronic stomach distress by my general practitioner in 2002. No warnings about dependence, addiction, or anything else. I took the medication for over 12 years, and when I finally learned of the complications that may come with withdrawal, I decided it was time to stop. Well, that might be simplifying it too much. I actually had a major melt-down, freaked out, and fell into a depression; and then I decided it was time to stop. I found a new doctor who had me wait six months to stabilize mentally before I tapered, which lasted for 18 months. Effective August 2018, I was four years benzo-free.

I had a varied collection of symptoms that have come and gone over the years. Some severe and even debilitating, others mild and annoying. They include severe anxiety, paresthesia (skin sensations), akathisia (inner restlessness), insomnia, heart palpitations, muscle tremors, tinnitus, benzo belly, flushing, slurred speech, hypersensitivity, and many more. These symptoms have entirely changed my life and put a strain on my marriage. I have been unable to work as a database programmer for almost a year now due to cognitive dysfunction and memory difficulties. I still have symptoms that come and go, but I am much better than I was, and I'm hopeful that one day I'll return to some semblance of a healthy life and be symptom-free.

You seem pretty open about what you went through.

I try to be as honest about myself as I can. And that includes when I write. If someone writes about a personal journey and doesn't put his or her true self into it, it doesn't ring true. Readers are smart. They know if your story is genuine or not. This is me, warts and all. Some of it's embarrassing. Some of it I'm not proud of. I'm an average guy lost in a crazy world just trying to figure the whole damn thing out. Trying to find my place. Trying to recover from this impossible illness. Perhaps, just perhaps, it lies in writing this book. Now wouldn't that be cool?

Why not a blog? Or a website?

I have nothing against blogs. I even tried writing one once, but it didn't take. It was a somber day when I decided to shut it down and disappoint both of my readers. Yes, both. And as for websites, I have one online now at www.BenzoFree.org that supplements this book and its findings. But still, for me, the book is the thing.

I love books. I love the detail that the format allows. I love the feel of the paper in my hands and to write notes in the margin with an actual pen and highlight sections in bright yellow. I love to take my time getting to know the writer and the story. I don't want to be hurried because I only have two minutes to read an article and I don't want 50 pop-up ads incessantly demanding my attention as I do. I want to relax and enjoy reading just as much as I enjoy writing.

So, you're old school.

Yeah, I guess so. And I'm kind of proud of it. I'm not an early adopter, nor do I really want to be. I don't have a Twitter account; I don't spend time on Instagram; I still can't get my mind around the real definition of a "meme." Seriously, what is a meme? "Anyone? Bueller? Bueller?"[3] Like I said, old school. I am fascinated by new technology and its benefits, but overall, I crave a slower pace of life and my experience with benzos solidified that desire. I'm not here to preach that my way of life is any better than the next because it isn't. It's just the one that works for me.

That's fair. So, will this book answer all my questions about benzos?

No. Are you kidding?

Even though finding information on benzo withdrawal can seem confusing at first, there is a ton of information available. Most of it's online. This book is focused on my experiences and research. I have my own opinions, and while I'll try to be as objective as I can in my presentation of the information, I won't always succeed. By nature, this book is limited. Don't confine yourself to one source for something as important as this. Educate yourself through multiple sources and be sure one of those is *The Ashton Manual*.

I've heard about *The Ashton Manual*. What is it?

The Ashton Manual's official title is *Benzodiazepines: How They Work and How to Withdraw*,[4] and it was written by Professor C. Heather Ashton DM, FRCP. It can be found online for free at www.benzo.org.uk/manual.

Prof. Ashton spent 12 years working with benzo recovery patients in her clinic. She is retired now but is praised by many as the world's leading expert on benzo withdrawal. No other resource has helped more people through this challenging experience. I can't tell you the number of times when I had a question or concern and went to her manual for help. I found her writing not only educational but reassuring and comforting. While her manual is full of medical facts and valuable information, she finds a way to let you know that she believes you can succeed and motivates you to do just that.

The Ashton Manual is THE guidebook for benzo withdrawal, end of story.

So how is your book different?

I am not trying to duplicate *The Ashton Manual*. I am not a medical expert like Prof. Ashton, and there is no way I would assume I could write anything as useful as her manual. This book is not a withdrawal guide. Instead, it's an informational resource about benzos and withdrawal with some personal insight from someone who has been through the experience first-hand.

What would you say is the most important factor in benzo withdrawal?

Mindset. Plain and simple.

Keeping a positive, balanced, and stable mindset throughout withdrawal was the hardest struggle of my life. The fear is relentless and maintaining confidence in my abilities to succeed was a constant battle. One that I failed at repeatedly. I know all too well that there are days when it's just not possible to stay positive or to stay calm. Days when you're mired in too much pain and hopelessness to even crawl out of bed. But most days don't have to be like that. There are ways to improve your chances for a successful experience.

Fear is enemy number one during benzo withdrawal. Fear causes anxiety, which causes symptoms, which causes more anxiety, which causes more severe symptoms, and on and on. But by developing tools to help stabilize our mental state along with sufficient preparation and education before taper, withdrawal can be a very manageable endeavor.

We'll talk more about this mindset in Part II of the book.

And who is your audience?

Anyone and everyone. I hope.

I know that this is a niche book and will only appeal to a limited percentage of the populace, and that's okay. My initial audience is obvious, people who are dependent on benzos and benzo-like drugs. I also want to focus on those who care for those people including spouses, family, friends, and even medical professionals. But I have a dream that even someone who has never heard of a benzo before might still find this book of interest and enjoy the read. It's my dream, and I'm sticking to it.

What are benzo-like drugs?

Benzodiazepines are a specific class of minor tranquilizers that are the central focus of this book. But there are similar classes of anti-anxiety drugs such as nonbenzodiazepines (z-drugs) and thienodiazepines that have the same dependence issues and withdrawal complications as benzos. When I speak of benzos in this book, I am usually including all these classifications unless otherwise stated. I'll elaborate more in chapter two.

What should I expect from you as an author?

You decided to take the time to read this book, and you have certain expectations. As you should. So, here's what you can expect:

Honesty - I'll be as honest, open, and forthright about my journey through benzo withdrawal as I can.

Objectivity - The benzo community is rife with its share of controversies. Much of the information we share with each other is conjecture based on personal experiences. Do I have opinions? Of course. Will they influence how I report things? At times, I'm sure they will. But, my goal is to be as objective as possible throughout and I will endeavor to make that happen.

Positivity - Most of us dealing with benzodiazepine withdrawal syndrome (BWS) have at times felt anger at doctors, pharmaceutical companies, or even the medication itself. It's completely understandable. But in this book, I try and leave most of that anger behind and focus more on positive change. I believe that working with doctors, and not against them, is the only path to true success.

Humor? - I've done my best to interject a little humor to lighten the mood, and a little humor is probably what you'll get.

How is the book structured?

Benzo Free is basically two books in one:

Part I - All About Benzos - The first part covers the science, culture, society, and other details about benzos and the world around them. It's chock full of information, and it might be of interest to anyone with a curious mind who wants to learn more about mental health and the role that benzos have played in that world.

Part II - All About Withdrawal - The second part is focused on the process of withdrawal. It combines facts and studies about benzo dependence, tapering, and withdrawal symptoms along with my own personal journey through this challenging period.

How you approach this book is up to you. Some may choose to read it cover to cover, and others may decide to use it more as a reference and jump to specific sections according to their interests and needs. I wrote the book with both methods in mind, and I hope that it is accommodating to your unique approach whatever that may be.

When do we get started?

How about now?

PART I
ALL ABOUT BENZOS

Introduction

Welcome to Part I of the book. Here is a brief rundown of the chapters:

- **Anxiety & Insomnia** – I'll start by talking about the history and current state of anxiety and insomnia in the world and treatment options for those disorders.
- **History & Science of Benzos** - This chapter is an introduction to benzos. A little about the history, a little about the science, and a variety of stats and facts thrown in just for fun.
- **Effects of Benzos** - Time to look at the effects of the drugs including their benefits, adverse effects, and even possible permanent effects.
- **Benzo Usage** - Who uses benzos? I'll examine street use, home use, and other especially vulnerable groups, like children and the elderly.
- **Benzos in the Media** - Benzos didn't become some of the best-selling drugs of all time without a bit of media help. In this chapter, I will take a peek at benzos in music, TV, movies, and celebrity culture.
- **Benzo Creators and Regulators** - Next, I'll look at who created these drugs and the regulations that govern the industry.
- **Benzos and the Law** - It's hard to talk about benzos without touching on litigation and our criminal justice system.
- **Other Benzo Stuff** - This is a bit of a grab bag. I'll discuss benzos in the environment and the economy, look at some of the leaders of the underground benzo community, and discuss primary goals for change.

It sounds like a lot. And it is. So, let's get going.

CHAPTER 1

ANXIETY AND INSOMNIA

Why start with a chapter on anxiety and insomnia?

Before I go into too much detail on benzodiazepines, I would be remiss if I didn't back up and talk a bit about the underlying ailments that yearn so earnestly for a quick and easy cure. Treating anxiety, insomnia, depression, and overall mental health is a constant struggle for so many medical professionals and patients. To better understand the world of benzos and the need that created the drug, we need to start with mental illness.

Mental Illness

Okay, I'll play along. How about the numbers? How many people are affected with mental health problems?

At some point, every one of us has had to deal with anxiety, depression, or some other form of mental health issue. It's a regular part of life. Unfortunately, some people are afflicted with this struggle more than others. We identify these people as having a mental health disorder. And these disorders can have some dire consequences.

For adults 45 years old and under in the year 2015, suicide was the third leading cause of death for U.S. women, the second leading cause of death for U.S. men,[5] and the number one cause of death for men in the U.K.[6]

Mental health disorders are a big problem.

What are the most common mental health disorders?

Conditions that fall under the mental health umbrella include anxiety, depression, PTSD, alcoholism, substance abuse, bipolar disorder, anorexia, bulimia, panic disorder, postpartum depression, schizophrenia, seasonal affective disorder, erectile dysfunction, insomnia, restless leg syndrome...the list goes on and on. The human brain is still the most complex computer on this planet and anything that complicated has its problems.

While the psychiatric community has come a long way in treating these conditions, they still have a long way to go. Too often, people don't seek help for mental conditions. Many don't have the resources available. Many are too afraid or too ashamed to reach out. Many who seek help are misdiagnosed, over-medicated, or don't follow up on their treatment. And if they do get prescribed a long-term medication, they can experience side effects, some severe enough that make the treatment worse than the cure.

On top of all that, mental health has an image problem.

Okay, I'll take the bait. What image problem?

Glad you asked! One of the key problems with mental illness is its innate invisibility. Remember the car accident analogy from the preface? I opened with that because I believe it helps call attention to this problem. We can see a broken leg. We can find cancer with an MRI. We can locate heart defects with an X-Ray. We can identify a thousand different maladies with a simple blood test. But when it comes to mental health, the waters get muddy. It's mostly subjective. Sometimes the patient can't articulate what is wrong. Sometimes the patient does, but he's misunderstood or misdiagnosed. And sometimes the patient isn't believed at all.

Sorry to be blunt, but aren't some people faking it? Exaggerating things? Using "mental illness" as an excuse?

That's a great question. And to be completely honest, a fair one too.

Yes, some people are faking it. With over seven billion people on this planet, the odds would be staggering to think that none of those people have ever faked, or at least exaggerated, an illness. In fact, I would journey to say that most of us have at least stretched the truth about an illness to say...take a sick day? How about to get out of a blind date? Or to excuse yourself from a boring meeting? We all have faked, or at least exaggerated, an illness. And mental illness is no different.

Unfortunately, most people are not faking it. It just doesn't make sense. Even though faking sickness can occasionally get you out of something you wish to avoid, or garner sympathy from a loved one, it comes with a vast array of disadvantages. Loss of job. Loss of freedom. Loss of love. Loss of respect. Loss of independence.

Medical science is just that: a science. Medical professionals are trained to be scientists. That works great when there is specific scientific evidence of a disease or injury. But when it comes to mental health, your doctor or therapist has one thing to go by: What you tell her.

The psychological sciences are inherently subjective. As patients, we can try to relay what it's like living within our minds, but it will never be an objective study of our brains. It can't be. We will exaggerate some things. We will underplay others. We will omit details that we think might not be pertinent. We are human, it's what we do. Most of us try to do our best, but we will never be able to ultimately share the experience of living with our "condition." And that leaves others in the dark when they try to help us.

Add to that the current health care system, which can be limiting for both patients and providers. The average time a doctor spends with a patient can be as low as seven minutes. It's ridiculous to think that a medical professional can get to know her patient in that amount of time. In psychiatry, an initial appointment is usually longer but still far too short to thoroughly understand the patient and her struggles. And in the end, that appointment often ends with a prescription. With psychology, things get better, and the counselor gets a chance to know his patient over time. But time is money, and it can get quite expensive.

Doctors are also bombarded with influence from pharmaceutical companies, trade magazines, medical organizations, and other sources who often have their own agendas. Sometimes, this influence affects your treatment.

It's Just Anxiety

What about anxiety specifically?

Those of us who suffer from chronic anxiety find it almost impossible to relate our experience to others. In Scott Stossel's brilliant book, *My Age of Anxiety*, the author opens with the following quote by Søren Kierkegaard from 1844. I have yet to find a better description of what it's truly like to live with chronic anxiety, so I must follow Stossel's lead and include it here.

> *And no Grand Inquisitor has such dreadful torments in readiness as anxiety has, and no secret agent knows as cunningly as anxiety how to attack his suspect in his weakest moment or to make alluring the trap in which he will be caught, and no discerning judge understands how to interrogate and examine the accused as does anxiety, which never lets the accused escape, neither through amusement, nor by noise, nor during work, neither by day nor by night.[7]*

What causes anxiety?

Anxiety is a normal human physiological, psychological, and emotional process often in response to a stressful situation. But I really can't go too far without talking a bit about fight-or-flight. So, let's start there.

The fight-or-flight response is a physiological response to perceived danger to prepare the body for either fighting or fleeing. When triggered, the body releases a cascade of epinephrine, norepinephrine, estrogen, testosterone, dopamine, and other stress hormones. These trigger reactions in the body including increased heart rate, breathing rate, muscle tension, and an increase in oxygenated blood to the larger muscle groups.

Now the body is prepared. It's prepared to survive. The only problem is, we don't experience true risk-of-life situations as much as we used to. The amygdala part of our brains, which triggers this fight-or-flight response, can't always identify a real threat from a perceived threat. And this response is often triggered when we really don't need it.

When the human race was in its infancy, our lives were simpler but also more dangerous. We spent most of our days seeking food, water, shelter, and warmth. We also spent time eluding danger. But things have changed. Few of us must face off a wild hippo just to get to the office in the morning.

That state of preparation...that state of readiness...that is called anxiety.

When does anxiety become a problem?

Even in our modern world today, anxiety is still a regular part of life. You might have felt it when that car almost hit you on 25th Street. Or perhaps when you wanted to ask that boy out to the dance. Or maybe when you were in the waiting room for your first acting audition or when that sudden turbulence hit mid-flight somewhere over Ohio. We experience some level of anxiety every day. For most people, it's a normal part of life, and it doesn't cause any long-term complications.

It becomes a problem when it becomes excessive. It becomes a problem when it becomes chronic, when it interferes with a healthy life or keeps you from doing things you want to do. For some, anxiety includes excessive worry, insomnia, chronic nervousness, panic attacks, stomach distress, muscle tics and tremors, heart palpitations, hot and cold flushes, depression, and even suicidal ideation. For some, anxiety is a life-altering condition. One, from which, they want nothing more than to escape.

Anxiety kills relatively few people, but many more would welcome death as an alternative to the paralysis and suffering resulting from anxiety in its severest forms.[8]

— David H. Barlow, *Anxiety and Its Disorders* (2002)

Are there specific types of anxiety disorders?

Let's look at the ones listed in the Diagnostic and Statistical Manual of Mental Disorders (DSM-IV-TR) provided by the American Psychiatric Association (APA).

The term "anxiety" can cover a wide range of psychological conditions from normal event-triggered anxiety like the fight-or-flight response, to a wide variety of short and long-term anxiety disorders. These can include Generalized Anxiety Disorder (GAD), Obsessive-Compulsive Disorder (OCD), and Post-Traumatic Stress Disorder (PTSD). There are also Simple, Social and Specific Phobias. Some of the disorders have less clever names like Acute Stress Disorder, Substance-Induced Anxiety Disorder, Adjustment Disorder with Anxious Features, and Anxiety Due to a General Medical Condition. Agoraphobia and Panic Disorder round out the list.[9]

What causes anxiety disorders?

Since there are so many different types of anxiety disorders and variations on each type, you might assume that there would be a wide array of causes — and you would be right. The number of theories on what drives certain people to develop excessive anxious behaviors is quite large and far too complex to list here. Still, science has come a long way and has identified many factors that play a role. Most of these theories fall into one of two camps: biological (genetic, brain chemistry, medical conditions) and environmental (stress, life events, childhood, trauma). Let's start with biological.

A unique study by Andy Morgan at the Yale School of Medicine discovered a key brain chemical called neuropeptide Y (NPY) that might be a factor. Discovered in 1982, NPY is a peptide in the brain involved in regulating diet, balance, and the stress response. Morgan studied U.S. Special Operations Forces trainees at Fort Bragg who were undergoing the famous SERE (Survival, Evasion, Resistance, and Escape) program. These aspiring SEALs and Green Berets are exposed to three weeks of extreme physical and psychological hardship to determine if they could withstand the stress of being a prisoner of war.[10]

Morgan made a startling discovery. The special forces recruits who performed the most effectively during SERE had significantly higher levels of NPY than the poorer performing recruits. As much as one-third higher. In fact, some individuals with high NPY levels seem utterly immune to developing post-traumatic stress disorder (PTSD). No amount of stress can break them.[11]

Another study published in the journal *Current Biology* uncovered physical changes in the brain. The study was conducted by the Weizmann Institute of Science in Israel and found that people with anxiety disorders see the world differently than others because emotional experiences induce plasticity in their brain circuits that last after the experience is over. The study noted that anxious individuals tend to over-generalize emotional experience, whether they're threatening or not, and that this reaction isn't something that an anxious person can control since it's a fundamental difference in the brain.[12]

According to Stossel, "the number of studies on heritability of anxiety is climbing into the tens of thousands, and the overwhelming conclusion of almost all of them is that your susceptibility to anxiety — both as a temperamental tendency and as a clinical disorder — is strongly determined by your genes."[13]

So, the cause of anxiety is biological?

Not so fast. Yes, there is a lot of evidence that anxiety disorders have a biological basis, but environmental factors also come into play. As with most things in life, the answer is not black or white, especially when considering something as complicated as the human brain. You have to leave some room for gray (pun intended).

Let's look back at the study with the U.S. Special Operations Forces. Even though they located a neuro-peptide that can identify some soldiers as almost immune to PTSD, that is not the case for most of us. Those with normal to above normal levels of tolerance for anxiety would still be hard-pressed not to develop PTSD after extreme life-events such as war, crime, natural disasters, or abuse.

You can also find evidence for environmental causes in traditional psychoanalysis. If I wrote the following dialog, "Tell me about your childhood" for a therapy scene of a screenplay, I would be ridiculed for using such a cliché. But, it's a cliché for a good reason. Events in our childhood can, and do, affect what we think, how we react, and how our psyche develops. We see it repeatedly. The effects of the over-bearing mother, the distant father, and the playground bully can leave life-altering scars on our mental and emotional state.

In the end, the answer is both. Anxiety disorders are caused by both biological and environmental factors. To help those suffering from these disorders we need to work at it from both sides.

I recently read an article about gut bacteria and anxiety. Do you know anything about this connection?

For years, researchers have known that the brain and the digestive system are closely linked. Most of the research in the past has been focused on our mind's effect on our digestive system, and not the other way around. Lately, though, the tables have been turned. The focus of these recent studies has been on inflammation in the gastro-intestinal tract and how that inflammation may affect our mental well-being.

Serotonin is often thought of as the hormone of happiness. While serotonin is chemically active in the brain, most of it is made in the intestinal tract. Therefore, there is an assumption among some scientists that inflammation, or a disruption in the health of the GI tract such as Inflammatory Bowel Syndrome (IBS), can affect a person's mood and mental stability.

Researchers in Ontario, Canada have been investigating intestinal bacteria and their effect on the human brain and mood.[14] Through research on laboratory mice, they have proven that bacteria in the gut can seriously affect mood. According to an article from the U.S. Office of Naval Research regarding the study, "They also were able to control the moods of anxious mice by feeding them healthy microbes from fecal material collected from calm mice.[15]" Kind of gross, I know, but the results were illuminating. Diversity of gut microbiota was found to be beneficial to the mice.

This and other studies have led many to believe that probiotic supplements for humans will help with mental wellbeing. That sounds logical, but it's jumping the gun a bit. We're not mice. More human studies need to be done. Also, we don't exactly know which probiotics are beneficial to humans even if this is the right direction. Still, it's promising news and perhaps a brand-new area of psychological study.

What are some short and long-term effects of anxiety?

The list of possible short-term effects is a lengthy one and includes dizziness, fatigue, muscle aches, nausea, and more. I could list them all here, but since the short-term effects mirror many of the symptoms of benzodiazepine withdrawal syndrome, I'll save that until later.

Long-term effects can include insomnia, early memory decline, increased risk of stroke, and a series of negative impacts at work, home, and all aspects of life.

What about benefits? Is there an upside to having anxiety?

Whew, I'm glad you asked that. I was getting depressed. Yes, there is.

People who worry a lot have a high level of activity in a part of the brain that responds to danger and threats. Perhaps the danger is real, and perhaps it's not, but that response just might keep the anxious person safe from threats that other people might miss. While the constant worrying might drive us nuts, it might also keep us out of harm's way.

For example, I have always had a mild to moderate fear of heights. When I went through benzo withdrawal that fear was significantly heightened. Mountain roads that used to be an easy drive now scare the crap out of me. In the past few months, it's gotten a bit better, but I still have a way to go to return to normal.

Anyway, the downside is that my fear of heights limits some of my activities. I avoid things I want to do purely out of fear. Still, while most of the time it's too restrictive, it does prevent me from doing foolish things like taking a selfie while balancing on a rock leaning over the rim of the Grand Canyon. Perhaps the rock will hold and perhaps it won't. I'm not going to take the risk, and the one time that it gives way, well, I won't be the idiot falling one thousand feet into the Colorado River.

Anxious people often respond to threats that don't really exist or overreact to minor threats. But that same behavior just might save our lives one day.

What about intelligence and creativity?

This is where it really gets good.

A simple term used for those of us with anxiety is "over-thinkers." Our minds are always working, constantly creating. Sometimes that creation is negative, obsessive, and hurtful to ourselves. Other times, not so much. Either way, our brains are continually dreaming up new ideas. Great theorems. Great songs. Great movies. Great discoveries. Great books. Great art. Whether the discovery is scientific, mathematic, artistic, or any other discipline, the link between anxiety, creativity, and intelligence is undeniable.

One of the greatest poets of the 19th century, Emily Dickinson, suffered from debilitating anxiety and was often housebound. Her suffering fed her creativity. She rarely left her bedroom after she turned the age of 40. Darwin was also housebound by his anxiety for decades and would probably never have been able to finish his work on evolution if it wasn't for this "disability." Sir Isaac Newton invented calculus, which no one knew about for ten years because he was too agoraphobic to leave his home. Michelangelo suffered from Obsessive-Compulsive Disorder (OCD). Vincent Van Gogh, F. Scott Fitzgerald, Nikola Tesla, and even Abraham Lincoln have battled anxiety.[16]

And pop culture is no different. Adele, Drew Barrymore, David Beckham, Kristen Bell, David Bowie, Ray Charles, Eric Clapton, Dick Clark, John Cleese, Cheryl Crow, Miley Cyrus, Paula Deen, Johnny Depp, Judy Garland, Whoopi Goldberg, Anthony Hopkins, Scarlett

Johansson, Ashley Judd, Demi Lovato, John Mayer, Marilyn Monroe, Sir Laurence Olivier, Bonnie Raitt, Mickey Rourke, Sarah Silverman, Howard Stern, Emma Stone, Amanda Seyfried, Joey Votto, and Oprah Winfrey have all had difficulties with anxiety and anxiety-related disorders. Quite a list, eh?

Some people say that anxiety isn't a real disease, that it's all in my head. They say that if I tried harder, I could be normal. How do you respond to them?

Some people view mental illness as a weakness of character. "Stop worrying. Stop thinking so much. Stop obsessing. Stop wallowing in your own misery. Just be positive. Think of happy things. Suck it up." I've heard all of these and so many others. My response to them: "Don't you think I would if I could?"

There is some element of truth in each of the statements above. "Be positive" is a good mantra. "Suck it up" is appropriate, in certain circumstances. "Stop worrying" is a great idea. The real disconnect here is not that these statements don't have some merit. Instead, it's in the level of difficulty it is for different people, with different thought patterns, nervous systems, histories, and genetics to successfully "stop worrying."

I suffer from anxiety. It comes and goes, but since I started withdrawal, it came on quite strong and has remained. If someone says to me "just stop worrying," I get a little offended. Not in the literal message itself, but more in its connotation. What I hear, right or wrong, is "why don't you just stop worrying? It's easy. I do it all the time. It's not that hard." And perhaps that is true for some. It's not for me. Humans don't all think alike. I have no idea what thoughts roam about in your head, and you have no idea what thoughts hang out in mine.

I have an active brain. Not only do I obsess on thoughts — especially negative thoughts — but I have physical repercussions from those thoughts. I am wired differently. So, while not obsessing about an upcoming event may be easy for one person, it's not for me. If they gave a Ph.D. in obsessing, I would have graduated summa cum laude. I obsess about everything.

I have a soft spot in my heart for animals, and if I see an animal being mistreated, I can worry for days even if there is nothing I can do. If I have an upcoming medical procedure, I've already thought through every possible complication and outcome, and I'm sure the worst one is going to happen. If my wife is late coming home, I'm sure she's been in an accident, and I'm in the car driving frantically looking for her. If my mom calls, I'm instantly worried that something has happened to her or my dad before I even hear her voice.

Trust me. I don't do this because it's fun. It sucks. I wish to hell it would stop. But this, in varying degrees, is how I've been my whole life. And it is a problem. Some years it's been mild and not a significant hindrance to my daily life. Other years, such as during benzo withdrawal, it can be debilitating.

How are people with anxiety treated?

As I discussed earlier, many view anxiety as weakness. Weakness of the human spirit. Weakness of the will. And this view is not new. In fact, in military history, it's quite prevalent.

British army deserters were put to death until World War II. In fact, British generals stated in reputable medical journals that men who panicked during combat should be sterilized, "because only such a measure would prevent men from showing fear and passing on to another generation their mental weakness." In the U.S., General Patton wanted combat exhaustion (war neurosis) to be punishable by death, claiming it was a mere "problem of the will."[17]

This view is not isolated to the military. In all walks of life, the confident and less anxious individual is celebrated while the rest are derided for being weak. Throughout history, people with anxiety have been humiliated, demeaned, shunned, incarcerated, and even killed. It's not a pretty picture.

And yet, anxiety and weakness really have nothing to do with each other. Few people would call the most decorated Olympian of all time as weak. And yet, Michael Phelps has dealt with severe anxiety and depression for years. Following the 2012 Olympics in London, he said, "I didn't want to be in the sport anymore...I didn't want to be alive anymore." He stayed in his room for almost five days barely sleeping or eating.[18]

In our books, movies, TV, video games, and general pop culture we celebrate the brave one, the hero, and condemn the weak. But perhaps the tide is turning. More and more celebrities, and even royals, are now speaking about their struggles with mental health issues as awareness is raised.

Do you wish people were more sensitive to your sensitivity?

Nicely phrased. We're all sensitive about something. We all have triggers. We're all human. Sure, it would be nice if everyone, you know, "got me." Who doesn't want that? Still, I don't really blame others too much. I must admit that as sensitive as I am to my issues, I am probably just as insensitive to theirs. We can't dress in a coat of bubble-wrap each time we go outside. It doesn't really protect us, and in the end, we just wind up looking at life through distorted plastic. Life is good and bad, exhausting and wonderful. You can't block out the bad without also blocking out the good. There must be a balance for each of us.

While I was going through benzo withdrawal, I came across a quote by Shantideva, a Buddhist monk who lived in the early 700s CE, which has become one of my all-time favorites.

> *Where is there enough leather*
> *To cover the surface of the Earth?*
> *But just having leather on the soles of one's feet,*
> *Is the same as covering the whole Earth.*[19]

Thanks to benzo withdrawal, I am more sensitive now then I have ever been in my entire life. And I wish to hell I wasn't. I don't enjoy being overly sensitive. Then again, I don't know anyone who does. I work hard being less reactive, and I am not asking for any special treatment or accommodations because of this condition. It's my burden, and I am the one who must learn to live with it. But it's real, despite what some may say, and I'm doing the best I can to manage it.

As for me, I'm cutting the leather and making shoes.

How many people suffer from anxiety? How big of a problem is it really?

It's big. Really big. According to the World Health Organization (WHO), 263 million people were living with anxiety disorders in 2015. That's about 3.6% of the world's population.[20] In 2017, it's estimated that depression and anxiety disorders combined cost the global economy about one trillion U.S. dollars each year in lost productivity.[21] Since less than half of the people who suffer from anxiety seek help, the real number is significantly higher.

Clearly, if you suffer from anxiety like me, you're not alone.

So, is the anxiety problem getting worse?

I wish I could say no.

"Between 2002 and 2006, the number of Americans seeking medical treatment for anxiety increased from 13.4 million to 16.2 million," according to IMS Health, the largest vendor of U.S. physician prescribing data.[22] That's a 21% increase in just four years. And the trend continued. Statistics from the National Health Service (NHS) reveal that British hospitals treated almost five times as many people for anxiety disorders in 2011 as they did in 2007, and they issued a record number of tranquilizer prescriptions[23] — most of which were probably benzos.

What do the statistics look like for children?

When we look at mental health in children, things do not improve.

Suicide for people 15–24 years old is now the third leading cause of death in the U.S. This number has tripled since the 1950s.[24] A National Institute of Mental Health study of millennials found that by the age of eighteen, 35% will be diagnosed with an anxiety disorder, 25% will be diagnosed with substance addiction, and 20% will have a behavioral disorder. Accounting for the overlap, one of these disorders will affect one in two young people.[25]

Many educators are very concerned about this trend. A psychologist at Weill Cornell Medical College, Robert Leahy, recently said in an article in *Psychology Today*, "The average high school kid today has the same level of anxiety as the average psychiatric patient in the 1950s."[26]

And unfortunately, the numbers don't improve when they get to college. In a 2009 survey by the American College Health Association, 46% of college students said they felt "things were hopeless" at least once in the previous 12 months, and "nearly a third had become so depressed that it was difficult to function."[27] Many professors and college health experts claim that students seem more fragile today than ever before and that this fragility has forced them to change their behavior in class, including their curriculum, to accommodate the heightened sensitivity of today's students.

What's causing the increase?

Many researchers are calling our modern era, "the age of anxiety." While biological causes might be shifting and causing part of the increase in anxiety rates, most researchers are focusing on environmental causes, or to be more specific, cultural pathology.

> *Our way of life promotes anxiety and its consequences. Anxiety makes us fearful. It makes us irritable and therefore easily — and excessively — prone to anger. Fear and anger are powerful antagonists to reason and reflection. They grab us by our primitive brain and urge us to "fight, flee or freeze." New media, social media and political leaders command our attention with outrage and alarm. The media's daily reminders to be very afraid and politicians' apocalyptic rhetoric reverberate throughout the Internet, keeping our anxiety at a constant high level.*[28]

— Renee Garfinkel, *The Washington Times*

Okay, can I just say a quick side note here? I wish I could write like Renee. "Apocalyptic rhetoric reverberate throughout the Internet..." That's good stuff.

How about a gender difference? Does anxiety affect women more than men?

It appears so. In 2015, according to the World Health Organization (WHO), 4.6% of females and only 2.6% of men had anxiety disorders.[29] The numbers are similar when we look at girls. According to the National Institute of Mental Health (NIMH), 38% of girls between the ages of 13 and 17 have an anxiety disorder, while only 26% of boys do.[30]

The causes for the discrepancy between the genders allows for some speculation. Some are obvious and may include societal expectations, changing gender roles, uneven domestic workload, hormonal changes, and generalized underlying fear for safety from unwanted advances or rape. There's also a possible evolutionary cause that relates to child-rearing. Since women have traditionally looked after the young, they're more attuned to danger that might threaten children.

There are some biological factors too. Some women in North America experience "estrogen dominance," a phenomenon where there is either too much estrogen or not enough progesterone for hormonal balance. Too much estrogen can cause irritability and anxiety symptoms, while progesterone has a stress-relieving and calming effect.

Social media is a factor here too. According to the Pew Research Center, social media use among women is at an all-time high: 73% of American women are active on social media outlets compared to 65% of men.[31] Also, women, and especially girls, are often more image conscious than men. In a 2010 study at Stanford University, girls aged eight to 12 were asked to surf the Internet for up to five hours, then describe how happy and socially comfortable they felt. The more time the girls spent online, the less content and at ease in social settings they became.[32]

Whether the cause is societal, hormonal, or technological, women are suffering from anxiety in high numbers and need help.

What about men? Aren't they affected by anxiety disorders too?

Of course, they are. While it may look like women take the brunt of anxiety's punishment, the gap is not as wide as it first appears. In fact, there might not be a gap at all. Anxiety in men is just as severe of a problem as it is in women, mostly because men are far less likely to seek help. As I mentioned earlier, suicide is the number one killer of men in the U.K. under the age of 45.[33]

"[Society] thinks men are doing pretty well ok compared to women," says Psychotherapist Damien Ridge, professor of health studies at the University of Westminster. He added, "When men talk about depression in their own terms, quite a large proportion are not doing so well."[34] Only 25% of people who seek help for depression in the U.K. are men, and yet recent studies suggest that the number of men dealing with depression is nearer 50%. Men are less likely to go to a doctor, and their upbringing and the shame associated with talking about or expressing feelings means they may not talk about it even if they do make it to their appointment.[35]

Men and women deal with stress, anxiety, and emotions differently, and that difference needs to be addressed so that everyone can get the help that they need.

Insomnia: The Reluctant Sandman

Enough about anxiety. What about insomnia?

Many people who have taken benzos have had no issues with anxiety at all and took the drug as a sleep agent. So, let's look at insomnia for a bit.

Basically, insomnia is sleeplessness. Habitual, chronic sleeplessness. Most sources agree that more than 30% of the U.S. population suffers from some type of insomnia. In fact, most people have experienced some patch of insomnia at some point in their lives. Perhaps renting the apartment right next to the train tracks, above the nightclub, under the tap-dancing studio, and across from the neon sign wasn't the best idea, now was it?

Some groups suffer more than others. Students suffer the most and are well known for "getting by" on just four or five hours per night. The next group to struggle with insomnia is adults from 40 to 55 years of age followed immediately by those 65 or older. I guess the time to get sleep is in your late twenties and thirties. I wish I would have known that earlier.

What are the effects of insomnia?

Sleeplessness can produce abnormal amounts of cortisol, which can create weight gain, high blood pressure, and heart damage. It can even create — get this — depression and anxiety. Insomnia also has many adverse effects on society and business. People who suffer from insomnia have a slower reaction time and therefore a higher risk of accidents. A Harvard study revealed that sleep issues in the U.S. account for more than 274,000 workplace accidents a year costing upwards of 31 billion dollars.[36]

How much sleep is enough?

This one is quite often debated. Before the turn of the twentieth century, we averaged about ten hours of sleep a night. Now, most people get about six or seven.

The National Sleep Foundation (NSF) released results of a two-year world-class study on sleep back in 2014. They came up with an ideal sleep range based on age groups. Their recommendations for sleep duration are listed below. Please note, these are average recommendations and vary from person to person.

Sleep Duration Recommendations from the NSF:[37]

- Newborn (0–3 months): 14–17 hours
- Infant (4–11 months): 12–15 hours
- Toddler (1–2 years): 11–14 hours
- Pre-School (3–5 years): 10–13 hours
- School Age (6–13 years): 9–11 hours
- Teen (14–17 years): 8–10 hours
- Young Adult (18–25 years): 7–9 hours
- Adult (26–64 years): 7–9 hours
- Older Adult (65 +): 7–8 hours

What are the causes of insomnia?

As with anxiety, the causes of insomnia are varied. These include stress, poor sleep habits, medications, medical conditions, caffeine, menopause, travel, pregnancy, genetics, and even technology. Let's look at those last two for a moment.

In 2017, an international team of researchers published the results of a study in *Nature Genetics*. In a sample of 113,006 individuals, the researchers found seven genes linked to insomnia.[38] Scientists have also identified a group of neurons that help us stay awake when we need to. This neural circuit in the brain controls wakefulness and could offer new treatments for insomnia.[39]

Recent studies have also shown that screen time before bed can be another factor. The blue light of LED screens tricks our brains into believing it's daytime by stopping the production of melatonin. So, playing that last game of *Candy Crush* on your iPad, or watching that last guest on Stephen Colbert, might not be the best trick for a restful night sleep.

The causes of insomnia are just as confusing and disperse as those for anxiety, but researchers are making great strides and getting closer to more answers.

Treatment Options

What about treatment?

As you've just learned, anxiety and insomnia are widespread in today's world. You've also learned about some of the causes of these chronic problems. But I haven't really talked about treatments. So, let's do that now before I move on.

The debate over treatments for mental illness is intense. There are so many people, on so many sides, arguing so many differing opinions. There appears to be a love/hate relationship with people's take on benzodiazepines, antidepressants, vitamins and minerals, cannabis, mindfulness, counseling, aromatherapy, acupuncture, and all the other possible choices. The question each of us wants an answer to is simple; how do I feel better? The answer is complicated.

Everyone is different, more so when it comes to mental health than in almost any other area. Some psych meds appear to work well for some people, but not for others. Many aren't any better than a placebo. Some people thrive in counseling, others can't last the first session, and others will never even try. Some people find mindfulness and meditation to be lifesavers, others can't sit still for two minutes. Some find that their faith in God is their saving grace, others don't believe a god exists. Some... and it goes on and on. We're all different, and odds are there will never be that one solution for us all.

But we want it. We want that one solution so desperately. We want that quick fix. With all our money and all our science, where the hell is that "magic pill?"

It doesn't exist. And most likely it never will. We are complex. Our brains are complex. Our world is complex. Our lives are complex. Why do we think there should be a simple solution for what ails each of us? There's not. But there is help. It may take work, but there is help.

Most of the treatments for anxiety and insomnia fall into four distinct buckets:

- Counseling
- Medication
- Diet and Supplements
- Alternative Therapies

What about counseling?

Counseling is the go-to treatment for mental illness. It has been around the longest and has had the most long-term success. Although the specifics and methodologies have changed over time, talk therapy has stood firm. CBT, DBT, ACT, MBCT, MET, EMDR, CMMI, CRA, IPT, and FFT are just a few of the acronyms used to define counseling techniques. It can be quite confusing.

The most critical step is to find a counselor who you feel comfortable with. It may take several tries, but that's okay. This is a long-term relationship, and it's worth getting it right.

And medication?

This one is why we're all here. Psych meds. You may have powerful feelings about psychiatric medication, especially benzos, and for a very good reason. Still, to do justice to this book, I want to try and be as objective as I can be about this subject. In fact, even after my experience with benzos, I'm not "anti-med" as so many have become. I believe that some medications are life savers. That even includes many psych meds.

Psychiatric medications are broken down into classifications such as antidepressants, antipsychotics, anxiolytics, depressants, stimulants, and antimanic agents. Benzodiazepines fall under the anxiolytic classification since they're anti-anxiety drugs. This is the group we will be paying very close attention to in the rest of this book. For now, though, I'll move on since this is just a brief introduction.

I guess the next one is diet and supplements. Right?

Very good. You follow instructions well.

I wish that some of the controversy would wane when we move into the next subject, but not so much. Some camps believe that vitamins and supplements are the keys to longevity and a healthy life. Others feel strongly that if you eat a healthy diet, then you don't need any supplements. And there are those that think that mental health has nothing to do with diet and supplements at all.

And Alternative Therapies?

This category has almost as many options as the others. It includes massage, acupuncture, Ayurveda, meditation, mindfulness, yoga, art therapy, music therapy, light therapy, animal-assisted therapies, self-help groups, and many more. Since alternative therapies are quite often separate from standard medical practice, they're also less tested. Still, times are changing, and more studies have been released with some surprising results.

Can we finally talk about benzos?

I guess you've waited long enough.

CHAPTER 2

HISTORY AND SCIENCE OF BENZOS

All About the Drug

Okay. Let's start basic. What are benzos?

The term "benzos" is short for "benzodiazepines," a class of psychoactive prescription drugs developed in the 1960s. Also called "anti-anxiety medications" or "minor tranquilizers," benzos were developed to combat a variety of issues including panic attacks, anxiety, insomnia, muscle spasms, and seizures.

Is BZD the same thing as benzos?

Yes. BZD is an acronym for benzodiazepine commonly used in medical literature and studies.

When I tell people about benzos, they often have no idea what I'm talking about. Why is that?

The truth is that they probably have heard of them. Benzos are marketed by the more recognized brand names of Xanax, Valium, Ativan, Klonopin, and others. Compared to those names, the term "benzodiazepine" might have a bit of trouble making headway in the media. Let's face it, the word "benzodiazepine" is not sexy. That's why I like "benzo." It's shorter, easier to say, and even has a bit of pizzazz. Among the benzodiazepine withdrawal community, the term "benzo" is the norm.

But you make a good point. When I tell people that I'm recovering from dependence to benzodiazepines, most people have no idea what I'm talking about. It surprises me regularly that the term "benzo" or "benzodiazepine" is not a part of the global lexicon. This class of drugs has been around for over 50 years, the number of people affected by benzos is shocking, and yet few know what they are.

It comes down to money and marketing, just like so many other things. Pharmaceutical companies spend billions of dollars advertising the names of their drugs so you won't forget them. Names like Advil, Tylenol, Lipitor, Viagra, Pepcid, Sominex, Vicodin, Ritalin, and yes, Xanax, have become part of the human dialog. "Benzo" is still an underground term used primarily by those of us who have become dependent on the drug.

You seem focused on the name. Why does that matter?

I'm no business major, but I do know that brand awareness is critical to any product's marketing campaign. This is the same when you're trying to get peoples' attention about a cause. There are over 40 benzodiazepine medications (including z-drugs), each with their own scientific names and variety of brand and generic names. This creates confusion. And confusion is deadly in a marketing campaign.

Even when I was pondering over the title of this book, I struggled with its name, *Benzo Free*. I love the title, but would it garner any attention? Anyone who doesn't know what a benzo is will skip right past it. I contemplated a title like "The Psychological and Physiological Odyssey of Withdrawal from Xanax, Ativan, Valium, Klonopin, Lunesta, Sonata, Ambien and Other Benzodiazepines, Z-Drugs and Thienodiazepines or Similar Anti-Anxiety Medication and the Science, History, and Culture that Created the Problem." But that seemed a bit excessive.

I'm trying to raise awareness about benzos, and without brand awareness, it's a more difficult journey. So, for the rest of this book, I am going to emphasize the term "benzos." I'll use it in the title of this book, on the Facebook page, and on the website. Perhaps it will help. Perhaps not. But I'm going to give it the old college try.

How many people are taking benzos?

According to IMS Health, 36 million people in the U.S. alone were taking anti-anxiety drugs in 2013.[40] This classification can include benzodiazepines, nonbenzodiazepines (z-drugs), and thienodiazepines. For benzodiazepines alone, according to the *American Journal of Public Health*, 13.5 million adults filled prescriptions in 2013.[41]

How many are on long-term prescriptions?

Most benzo prescriptions are for short-term use. This is good since many governmental agencies and medical associations recommend that benzos not be prescribed for longer than two to four weeks. Unfortunately, despite the recommendations and warnings, at least five million people in the U.S. and U.K. alone are estimated to be on benzos long-term and have the potential for withdrawal complications.[42]

What are the most common anti-anxiety drugs?

Let's look at each class of drug:

Benzodiazepines - The most common benzodiazepines, starting with the most popular, are alprazolam (Xanax), lorazepam (Ativan), clonazepam (Klonopin), diazepam (Valium), and temazepam (Restoril).[43] Other common ones include chlordiazepoxide (Librium), clorazepate (Tranxene), estazolam (ProSom), and triazolam (Halcion).

Nonbenzodiazepines (z-drugs) - As for z-drugs, they include eszopiclone (Lunesta), zaleplon (Sonata), zolpidem (Ambien), and zopiclone (Zimovane).

Thienodiazepines - Thienodiazepines include bentazepam (Thiadipona), brotizolam (Lendormin), clotiazepam (Clozan), and etizolam (Depax).

Can you list all the benzos?

I have provided a list of benzodiazepines, z-drugs, and thienodiaz-epines in the appendix. This list also includes some basic information including their brand and generic names, market focus, onset, half-life, and potency.

Is there a difference between them?

Yes. The different benzos vary by four primary classifications: potency, speed of effectiveness, half-life, and focus of treatment. For example, Chlordiazepoxide (Librium) is better for alcohol with-drawal, midazolam is often used as anesthesia, and lorazepam (Ativan) is effective at controlling seizures.

When withdrawing, perhaps the most essential difference is that of potency. The second generation of benzos (Xanax, Ativan, Klonopin, Halcion) can be significantly more potent than the first generation (Valium). For example, 1 mg of clonazepam (Klonopin) is equal to 20 mg of diazepam (Valium). This is a critical factor to remember if you are tapering off your medication.

We'll learn more about these differences in the following chapters.

What are they prescribed for?

Benzos have a variety of therapeutic actions but can be broken down into five primary categories that Prof. Ashton described in her manual. These include anxiolytic (relief from anxiety), hypnotic (improving sleep), myorelaxant (muscle relaxation), anticonvulsant (relief from convulsions), and amnesiac (loss of memory, single-use for medical procedures).[44]

Are benzos effective?

They can be. At least in the short-term. I wouldn't be writing this book if the drugs weren't somewhat effective. The immediate effects of most benzodiazepines can make a person feel relaxed and some-times sleepy. Even a mild sense of euphoria. And many studies show that occasional, short-term use of benzodiazepines is effective for specific purposes including surgical procedures, alcohol withdrawal, and seizures.

What's the downside?

Well, that's a loaded question. I just might take the rest of the book to answer that one. But before we move on to that, I think it's important for us to learn more about the drug itself.

The History of Benzos

When did this whole benzo thing start?

Well, I could go all the way back to 3400 B.C. Seriously. Maybe not benzos per se, but mind-altering drugs do go back a long, long time. According to the U.S. Drug Enforcement Administration (DEA), the earliest reference to opium growth and its use is in 3400 B.C. when opium poppy was cultivated in lower Mesopotamia.[45] Benzodiazepines started a little bit later, somewhere around the mid-20th century AD.

The history of benzos may appear dry on the surface when you think of all the science and studies and science and medical jargon and science and politics and science and — well, you get the picture. But it's not dry. It's actually a pretty good story. It has ups and downs, twists and turns, politics, celebrity, drama, you name it.

So, get comfy and let me tell you the story of benzos, or at least part of it. Let's start in the 1950s with Leo Sternbach.

Who is Leo Sternbach?

Leo Sternbach was born on May 7th, 1908 in the town of Opatija in western Croatia.[46] He and his younger brother Guisi spent their days dreaming of life without the struggles of —

Wait a minute. Do I really need to know about his childhood?

No, I guess not. Let's jump ahead 25 years.

Krakow, Poland. 1931. Leo receives his doctoral degree in organic chemistry from the Jagiellonian University where he started working on a chemical group called the heptoxdiazines. Trust me, this is relevant. In 1941, he moved to the United States and joined the pharmaceutical firm Hoffmann-La Roche in New Jersey.[47]

Is that a better pace?

It's an improvement, but what does this have to do with benzos?

Wow. Short attention span, huh? I'll speed it up.

It was the 1950s, right about the time of *Mad Men*, if that helps create a visual backdrop and mood. Leo's bosses at Hoffman-La Roche wanted to find a better tranquilizer, and they assigned him to the task. Barbiturates had become infamous for dependence and addiction and the drug companies needed to find a safer alternative.

Leo remembered the chemical group he worked on in Krakow — you remember, the heptoxdiazines — and he wondered what would happen if he modified them a little? He tried over 40 different versions in animal testing, but none of them seemed to work. The company abandoned the project.[48]

In 1957, a research assistant came across a powder named Ro#5–0690 that had been synthesized a year earlier but was never tested. Without much thought, Sternbach sent it out for testing. "We thought that the expected negative result would complete our work with this series of compounds and yield at least some publishable material. Little did we know that this was the start of a program which would keep us busy for many years," said Sternbach.[49]

Later that year, Ro#5–0690 was found to have hypnotic and sedative effects similar to meprobamate (Miltown).

What's Miltown?

In 1954, the first real medication for anxiety hit the American market. It was called meprobamate and marketed as Miltown by Wallace Laboratories. By 1957, doctors had written 36 million prescriptions. There was no competition back then. It was the only tranquilizer on the market, and it did very well. More than a billion of these "peace pills" had been manufactured by 1957.

According to the *Newsweek* article "America's Long Love Affair with Anti-Anxiety Drugs,"[50] people weren't as cynical back in the 1950s. Following closely on the heels of Thorazine's big success in treating schizophrenia, some people referred to Miltown as "psychiatry's penicillin." Due to the stress of the Cold War, one civilian-defense film urged patriotic citizens to stash a bottle of tranquilizers in their fallout shelters.

Unfortunately, meprobamate had a few problems. In addition to its anxiolytic and hypnotic effects, it also had this nasty little side-effect of physical dependence. In fact, sudden withdrawal from the medication caused dangerous withdrawal symptoms. If someone wanted to stop taking Miltown, they had to taper from the drug very slowly. Does any of this sound familiar?

Miltown was heavily marketed to housewives, and it did exceptionally well. By the 1960s, though, another class of drugs came onto the market, and Miltown quickly faded from favor.

Was this new drug a benzo?

Very good. You're paying attention.

So, getting back to Leo Sternbach. Even though Ro#5–0690 is a very catchy name, they decided it needed something with more sizzle. But since they're chemists, they weren't very creative. Starting out as methaminodiazepoxide, the drug was eventually changed to chlordiazepoxide, which it's still called today. This new substance combined a benzene ring of atoms with a diazepine ring of atoms — yes, you guessed it, the very first benzodiazepine was born.

On February 24, 1960, the FDA approved the drug. It was officially released to the public after brief clinical tests at the University of Texas, even though some twenty thousand people had already been administered it.[51] "Controlled trials were not required for evaluation, and 'efficacy' was demonstrated by anecdotes and testimonials,"[52] stated A. Byrne in the journal *Australian Family Physician*. Hoffmann-La Roche called the drug Librium, derived from the word "equilibrium." And so, started the era of benzos.

Librium was considered safer than barbiturates since there were fewer side effects and fewer deaths from overdose. When Librium hit the market, it quickly outsold barbiturates and soon became the most prescribed drug in America. It remained that way until 1969 when it was replaced by another, perhaps better-known benzo: Valium.[53]

Ah, Valium. Now we're getting somewhere. Continue.

Thank you. I will.

Leo Sternbach didn't retire after the release of Librium. He kept working to find newer, better versions of benzodiazepines. In 1963, Hoffmann-La Roche released a brand-new benzodiazepine: diazepam. The company named it Valium, from the Latin "valere," meaning "to fare well" or "to be healthy." Ironic? Valium was 2 1/2 times more potent than Librium,[54] and just like its predecessor Miltown, it was heavily marketed to housewives. In 1966, the Rolling Stones released a song titled "Mother's Little Helper" that both celebrated and derided this medical breakthrough and its effect on the anxiety-prone suburban homemaker.

How long did Valium's reign last?

Quite a while.

Valium was the top-selling drug in the U.S. for 13 years, between 1969 and 1982. In the 1970s, the drug companies encouraged doctors to prescribe benzodiazepines instead of barbiturates through a campaign called CURB. It was so successful that by 1978 Valium became the most commonly prescribed drug in the entire world. In fact, there was even a suggestion that Valium should be added to drinking water, you know, like fluoride.[55]

As benzos became increasingly popular, a backlash also gained momentum. Scott Stossel shares his perspective on the growing movement in his book *My Age of Anxiety.*

> *By the middle of the 1970s, the FDA had collected numerous reports of benzodiazepine dependence...Many patients who had been on high dosages of Valium or Librium for long periods of time would experience excruciating physical and psychological symptoms when they stopped taking the medication: anxiety, insomnia, headaches,*

tremors, blurred vision, ringing in the ears, the feeling that insects were crawling all over them, and extreme depression — and, in some cases, seizures, convulsions, hallucinations, and paranoid delusions.[56]

Sounds like fun, doesn't it? In 1979, U.S. Senator Ted Kennedy led a Senate subcommittee hearing into suspected dangers of benzodiazepines where he said, "If you require a daily dose of Valium to get through each day, you are hooked, and you should seek help."[57] The backlash started, and drug companies were frantic to find something new.

The backlash increased in the '80s. Long-term benzo users were suffering from severe withdrawal symptoms, and the media picked up their stories. The Chief Medical Officer in the United Kingdom warned that long-term use of benzodiazepines caused or aggravated depression and increased suicidal tendencies. Several patients sued, but they were mostly unsuccessful.[58]

What was next?

Well, the drug companies needed to find something to replace benzodiazepines — and they did. A new class of anti-depressant drugs called Selective Serotonin Reuptake Inhibitors, aka SSRIs, was created. In 1987, Prozac entered the market and ousted benzos as the most popular drug for depression and anxiety.

I'm guessing that wasn't the end for benzos though, was it?

If it were, this book would be a hell of a lot shorter.

The pharmaceutical companies had another problem: What do you do when the drug that replaced the medication that had withdrawal issues has withdrawal issues of its own? Well, you could create a brand-new drug, or even better, release the old class of drugs all over again, but this time make them even stronger.

Okay, I know that sounded a bit cynical. Objectivity can be an uphill battle. I'll try harder.

In 1981, pharmaceutical manufacturer Upjohn (now part of Pfizer) released alprazolam, and they marketed it under the catchy name of

Xanax. While still a benzodiazepine, Xanax represented this new group of benzos that are even more potent than the ones in the 70s. Xanax is 20 times more potent than Valium.

By 1986, Xanax had overtaken Miltown, Librium, and Valium to become the best-selling drug in history. And by 2013, prescriptions for benzos in the U.S. climbed to 5.6% of the population.[59] The market demand for general anxiety medications was valued at $3.2 billion in 2014 and is expected to rise to $3.7 billion by the end of 2020.[60] Benzos were back and with a vengeance.

Thus endeth our tour through benzo history. Thank you for your time and attention. Please remember to fill out the survey on your clipboards.

Stats and Facts

That was almost interesting. How many people use benzos today?

Cool, stats. I love stats.

Before I dig deeper, though, I must voice a word of caution. Stats, just like anything else, can be misleading. Studies and statistics vary based on their sources, methods of collection, and yes, unfortunately, observational bias. There are also rare errors in the articles, documents, and websites themselves. And on top of all that, scientific studies within psychology and psychiatry can be inherently subjective since they rely on us, the patients, to tell them how we feel.

That is why I would continuously face conflicting numbers and outcomes as I was researching this book. I have attempted to report the most accurate information that I could, but please understand that my numbers are only as good as my sources, my limited medical research experience, and unfortunately, even my own personal bias — which I'll try diligently to keep in check but will occasionally fail in the attempt. So, back to the numbers.

How's this? The number of adults purchasing benzos increased from 8.1 million to 13.5 million in a span of 18 years, from 1996 to 2013. This was a 67% increase. Anxiety was the reason for 56% of the prescriptions, 12% for mood disorders, and 12% for unclassified (includes insomnia). Even more important, the overdose death rate involving benzodiazepines in that same 18-year period increased from 0.58 deaths to 3.14 deaths per 100,000 adults.[61] That is an increase of more than 500%.

According to IMS Health, the total number of U.S. adults taking anti-anxiety drugs in 2013 was over 34 million.[62] This number is significantly higher than the amount stated above for 2013, partially because it analyzes all anti-anxiety medications including benzodiazepines, z-drugs, and others. Let's break their information down a bit...

Total number of people in the U.S...[63]

- Taking psychiatric drugs: **79 million**
- Taking antidepressants: **41 million**
- Taking anti-anxiety drugs: **36 million**
- Taking ADHD drugs: **10 million**
- Taking antipsychotics: **7 million**

Total number of people in the U.S. taking anti-anxiety medication who are...[64]

- 5 years old or younger: **727,304**
- 6–12 years of age: **790,149**
- 13–17 years of age: **650,273**
- 18–24 years of age: **1,660,953**
- 25–44 years of age: **8,944,200**
- 45–64 years of age: **14,439,465**
- 65+ years of age: **9,691,791**

How much is this costing us?

Let's look at the U.S. Medicare System, the United States' health insurance program for those over 65. In 2012, the prescription program for Medicare didn't pay a dime for benzodiazepines since they were excluded from Medicare Part D. Then in 2013 after Congress overturned that ruling under pressure from patient groups and medical societies, Medicare started covering benzodiazepines. That first year it paid for nearly 40 million prescriptions costing more than $377 million to the government.[65]

What are the numbers in other countries?

In October 2012, *The Times* in Britain ran a front-page story titled "The Tranquiliser Trap: Scandal of 1 Million Hooked on Benzodiazepines." The article stated, "Doctors are still writing more than 11 million prescriptions a year for 'benzos' three decades after being encouraged to curtail their use."[66] In 2015, that number rose to 12 million.[67]

What about long-term use?

Determining the number of people using benzos on a long-term basis is a bit more difficult, but after everything is considered it's easy to guess that the total long-term users worldwide is in the millions.

According to *The Irish Times*, it's estimated that there are up to 1.5 million in Britain and up to four million in the U.S. who are on long-term prescriptions for benzodiazepines.[68] That's over five million people in the U.S. and U.K. alone where benzos are recommended for short-term use only.

Do most of the prescriptions come from psychiatrist offices?

No. And that's part of the problem. According to the National Institutes of Health (NIH), primary-care doctors prescribe 90% of all benzodiazepines.[69]

> *Doctors love prescribing benzos because it's the most efficient way to get a complaining patient out of the office in the shortest possible time. The patient is very satisfied at the moment, but may go on to develop a devastating addiction...90 percent of benzo prescriptions are written, often carelessly, by primary care doctors, who can spend only seven minutes with the patient without giving serious thought to the considerable risk of addiction.[70]*

— Dr. Allen Frances

The Science Behind Benzos

Okay, enough stats for now. Could you help me understand the drug better? What really are benzos?

I mentioned this briefly in the introduction, but let's recap here.

Benzodiazepines are a group of psychoactive drugs focused on treating anxiety, insomnia, and other related disorders. They're often classified as anti-anxiety medications or minor tranquilizers. Their name is derived from the chemical composition that combines a benzene ring and a diazepine ring.

This section of the book is about to get very technical. It took me days of reading and re-reading various articles to even start to understand it. If the science of how benzos work within the human body is not of interest to you, then please feel free to skim or even skip this section and jump ahead. I won't tell anyone, I promise. On the other hand, if you love science or are just curious by nature like me, then dive right in. Just remember, I warned you.

I want to know. Tell me how they work?

Well, that's where it gets a bit fuzzy. We have learned a lot, but there are still many unanswered questions. The human brain is complicated. Extremely complicated. We really don't know entirely how benzos interact with it. Our understanding of the mechanisms of benzodiazepines can differ based on various research studies and theories. This is incredibly frustrating for the scientists — and even more so for the patients taking the drugs.

The brain is complicated. Did I already say that? Sorry, but it's true. The brain is still the most complicated machine on this earth. In his book *When the Air Hits Your Brain: Parables of Neurosurgery*, neurosurgeon Frank Vertosick, Jr. put it this way:

> *The human brain: a trillion nerve cells storing electrical patterns more numerous than the water molecules of the world's oceans.*[71]

There is so much we have learned about the human brain, but still, so much more we have yet to discover. Its complexity leaves our

researchers and scientists with one nagging, recurring question —
how do we treat something we don't fully understand?

Medical necessity and business interests are reluctant to wait until
we have a complete understanding of the brain and nervous system.
Therefore, we move forward and develop theories, experimental procedures, and test new medications even when we have no clue how
that medicine did what it does.

When Leo Sternbach discovered the first benzodiazepine back in
the 1950s, he did so almost by accident. I'm sure he was a superstar at
the pharmaceutical firm of Hoffmann-La Roche because this new class
of drugs, these minor tranquilizers, sold like nothing they'd ever seen
before. And that's all well and good, but there was one nagging question.

How do they work?

**Why is that so important, though? They work. Isn't that good
enough?**

Pharmaceutical companies are required to do a series of tests on
new medications before they get approved for public use. Whether
this system of testing is thorough enough is of constant debate, but
even if their trials are adequate, there's still one thing that they most
likely wouldn't be able to do. Since the economic pressure to release
a new drug is so intense, no pharmaceutical company can take the
time to test for long-term side effects and complications. It would take
years, even decades. It's just not feasible, financially speaking.

Now, if we have some semblance of an idea as to the mechanism
of a particular drug, we can guess at any long-term effects. It's not
great, but it's something. But what about drugs for which we only have
limited knowledge of how they work? What about benzodiazepines?
How could anyone even remotely have said that these drugs were safe
when they didn't even understand how they work?

It's been 58 years. Why haven't they done more studies?

They have. But they are limited. During the past half-century since
benzos first were released, we have learned some vital information.

We have theories, and some consistency has evolved from research. But unfortunately, we still have many unanswered questions.

Part of the problem is funding. Most of the testing and studies performed on pharmaceuticals is paid for by the pharmaceutical companies themselves before the release of a new medication. Unfortunately, there is no incentive for these same companies to do any studies after a drug is released. Why would they? That usually leaves the government with the responsibility for research and with competition for tax dollars and consistent cut-backs of funding, research studies are limited. Anyway, I'm getting into politics here, back to the science.

Here's the thing. I am not a neurologist, neurobiologist, neuropathologist, or anything remotely starting with neuro and ending in -gist. So, I am approaching all of this as a layman. Bear with me.

I feel like you're eluding the question. How about I be more specific? I've heard that benzos work by affecting the GABA receptors. Is this true?

For the most part, yes.

It wasn't until the late 1970s, almost 20 years after the first benzodiazepine was released, that neuroscientist Erminio Costa discovered what was believed to be the salient chemical mechanism of benzodiazepine action. He identified benzos effect on a neurotransmitter called gamma-aminobutyric acid, or GABA as it's more often referred.

Let's start with Prof. Ashton's description from *The Ashton Manual* and then we can break it down to understand this better.

> *All benzodiazepines act by enhancing the actions of a natural brain chemical, GABA (gamma-aminobutyric acid). GABA is a neurotransmitter, an agent which transmits messages from one brain cell (neuron) to another. The message that GABA transmits is an inhibitory one; it tells the neurons that it contacts to slow down or stop firing. Since about 40% of the millions of neurons all over the brain respond to GABA, this means that GABA has a general quietening influence on the brain...*[72]

Okay, now we're getting somewhere. Can you simplify?

Sure. Let's try this definition from Wikipedia:

> *Benzodiazepines enhance the effect of the neurotransmitter gamma-aminobutyric acid (GABA) at the GABA receptor, resulting in sedative, hypnotic (sleep-inducing), anxiolytic (anti-anxiety), anticonvulsant, and muscle relaxant properties.*[73]

Still a bit long. Try again.

Okay. I think my favorite, although over-simplified, is from the Government Health System in New South Wales, Australia.

> *Benzodiazepines slow down the workings of the brain and the central nervous system.*[74]

There we go. Now, that's what I'm talking about.

I think the best way to really understand the mechanisms of benzodiazepines on the body is to break it down into terms. Let's start with the neurotransmitters: GABA and Glutamate.

I like where you're going with this, but first, can you define neurotransmitters?

Sure. I like to think of neurotransmitters as the pony express of the Central Nervous System. Too old school? How about this? Neurotransmitters are the Twitter of the Central Nervous System. Any better? These chemicals transmit messages between nerve cells, or neurons. They're the messengers. There are many types of neurotransmitters, and each of them has a different effect. You may have heard of serotonin, dopamine, and norepinephrine. But others like GABA and glutamate might not be as well-known, unless you're going through benzo withdrawal, of course.

Got it. So, back to GABA and Glutamate. What are they and what's the difference?

This is my favorite definition from a website called AddictionBlog.org:

> *Think of glutamate as the gas pedal: it excites things into action. GABA, on the other hand, puts on the brakes.*[75]

Perhaps it's not quite that simple, but it's a great start. When it comes to brain communication, there are two opposing systems: glutamate and GABA. Glutamate stimulates, and GABA inhibits. Together they regulate the level of excitability in the brain.

Tell me more about glutamate.

Glutamate is the most abundant neurotransmitter in the entire nervous system. It stimulates the neurons making them fire and helps brain development including learning and memory. Too much glutamate has been linked to Alzheimer's disease, stroke, Parkinson's disease, multiple sclerosis, and other diseases. Low levels of glutamate are often found in people with depression, schizophrenia, and autism. High concentrations of glutamate in the body can be toxic to nerve cells. If this happens over a prolonged period, it can cause damage, which is known as excitotoxicity.

And GABA?

GABA is the primary inhibitory neurotransmitter in the brain. GABA produces a general calming effect on your central nervous system by settling down nerve cells that get over-excited. When your neurons get over-excited, you get anxious. The more GABA, the calmer you feel. About 40% of the neurons in the brain respond to GABA,[76] which manages the influx of chloride ions through ligand-gated chloride channels called GABA(A) receptors.[77] Don't worry, that won't be on the test.

What's the difference between GABA and GABA receptors?

GABA is the chemical, the neurotransmitter. GABA receptors are the part of the neuron that can receive GABA neurotransmitters. So, only neurons with GABA receptors can be influenced by the calming effect of GABA, and if those receptors ever become damaged, then the nerve cells may not receive the calming message.

So where do benzos come in?

Benzos enhance the actions of GABA. Meaning, benzos increase the inhibitory effect of GABA on the neurons, therefore calming the brain and central nervous system.[78] For this reason, benzodiazepines have been found useful in treating anxiety, insomnia, muscle spasms, epilepsy, alcohol detoxification, and is helpful in certain medical procedures.

Okay. So, benzos increase the effect of GABA, which calms you down. That's not too complicated.

Hold on. That's not quite the whole story. You didn't think it would be that easy, did you? GABA does seem to get all the press when it comes to benzos, but it's not the complete picture.

...benzodiazepine actions are by no means confined to a particular neurotransmitter or brain pathway.[79]

— Prof. Ashton

Prof. Aston's paper titled "Protracted Withdrawal Syndromes from Benzodiazepines," published in 1991, is a great resource here. In that paper, she notes that GABA inhibits both the nervous activity in the brain and the release of excitatory neurotransmitters such as acetylcholine, noradrenaline, dopamine, and serotonin. The clinical effects of benzos are most likely a result of a combination of these reactions.[80]

Make sense?

Kind of. You mentioned dopamine. I know that one's a factor in addiction. What does it have to do with benzos?

Just like GABA and glutamate, dopamine is a neurotransmitter. The effect that dopamine has on the receiving neurons depends on its source, destination, type, and role. Dopamine is a big player, and just like the brain, it's complex. Dopamine is responsible for a lot of our emotions, desires, and motivation including the initiation of muscle movement.

Dopamine is a neurotransmitter that helps control the brain's reward and pleasure centers.[81]

— Psychology Today

Dopamine is also a big player in addiction. All abused drugs including heroin, cocaine, and alcohol increase dopamine in one way or another. And this includes benzos, but I'm getting ahead of myself again. I came across a study at the University of Geneva, Switzerland lead by Dr. Christian Luscher that looked at benzos to identify the point of convergence for all neurobiological pathways to drug addiction. They were trying to find the common mechanism. Their results suggest that this commonality is when dopamine surges in response to taking one of these addictive drugs that initiates a change in the plasticity in dopamine-producing cells.[82]

As I discussed earlier, addictive drugs increase the levels of dopamine in the system. It turns out that benzos are no exception. Benzodiazepines increase the firing of dopamine neurons in the ventral tegmental area of the midbrain. This is an area of the brain that is ripe with dopamine and serotonin neurons. They do this through positive modulation of GABA(A) receptors in nearby interneurons. This disinhibition triggers drug-evoked synaptic plasticity in excitatory afferents onto dopamine neurons and underlies drugs reinforcement.[83]

Did you get that?

Seriously? I think my brain is going to explode. Try again.

I didn't understand it the first time I read it either. Nor the third, fourth, or fifth. Let me see if I can make sense of it for both of us. Here are two key terms to keep in mind as I describe the mechanism:

- **Inhibitory neurons (GABA)** produce GABA neurotransmitters, primarily influenced by alpha-1 GABA subtype.
- **Dopaminergic neurons (DA)** produce dopamine neurotransmitters, primarily influenced by alpha-3 GABA subtype.

For this scenario, we're going to look at the ventral tegmental area (VTA) of the midbrain. There are two types of neurons, inhibitory neurons (GABA) and dopaminergic neurons (DA), that I want to look at here. Not only do these two types of neurons produce neurotransmitters, but they also receive neurotransmitters. Make sense so far? I'll pretend you said "yes."

Now it gets a bit more confusing. Both the GABA and DA neurons have GABA receptors, which means they can receive signals from the GABA neurotransmitters. But, these receptors are not precisely the same. There are two types of GABA(A) receptors that come into play here. The inhibitory (GABA) neurons are largely influenced by the alpha-1 subtype of GABA(A) receptors, and the dopaminergic (DA) neurons are largely influenced by the alpha-3 subtype. So, to clarify a bit, both the GABA and DA neurons have GABA(A) receptors, but they're affected by different subtypes.

Hang with me, now. This is where benzos come into the picture. Current benzodiazepines interact strongly with alpha-1 GABA(A) receptors on the inhibitory (GABA) neurons, therefore inhibiting the release of GABA. But benzos don't interact strongly with alpha-3 GABA receptors — the ones on the DA neuron. So, current benzos have little, if any, direct effect on dopamine release.

But they do have an indirect effect. Since benzos decrease the amount of GABA neurotransmitters released, there are less GABA neurotransmitters for the DA neurons to receive. And, since GABA is an inhibitory chemical, then the DA neurons receive less instruction to slow down the release of dopamine.

So, at the end of this fun science-class experiment, we learn that while benzos don't directly tell DA neurons to increase dopamine, they do influence its production through reduction in GABA.[84] Cool, eh?

And what about glutamate?

Drug addiction has been found to cause long-lasting changes in the human reward system including the migration of certain types of AMPA receptors — called GluA2-lacking receptors — from the interior to the surface of the dopamine-producing neurons.[85] The result is that these cells become susceptible to stimulation by...any guesses?

Glutamate?

Excellent. So, you are following this.

Not really, but continue anyway.

Okay. Well, Dr. Luscher and his Swiss colleagues showed that benzos induce AMPA receptor migration via the alpha-1 GABA(A) receptors. In their final experiment, the researchers recreated stimulated neuron firing in bursts like those produced by addictive drugs.

So, what does this mean?

Researchers have established that benzodiazepines behave similarly to other addictive drugs and leave lasting changes in the brain.

> *This was a nail-in-the-coffin study... Even if you clear the [benzodiazepine] drug from the body, there are long-lasting changes in brain architecture.*[86]

— Dr. Christian Luscher

Are you good now?

Not even close, but can we move on anyway? I'm starting to get a headache.

Me too. We'll revisit this science in Part II when we discuss the mechanics of benzodiazepine withdrawal syndrome (BWS). Until then, let's give our brains a break and look at the various types of benzos.

Different Types of Benzos

Great. How many different types of benzodiazepines are there?

There are about 40 different types of benzodiazepines on the world market today and another eight thienodiazepines and z-drugs.

Can you tell me more about the z-drugs?

Nonbenzodiazepines, or z-drugs, are often prescribed as an alternative to benzodiazepines. The nickname "z-drugs" came from the name of the drugs themselves; zolpidem, zopiclone, and zaleplon.

Nonbenzodiazepines were released in the late 1980s as an alternative to benzodiazepines. They have entirely different chemical structures to benzodiazepines, and yet they have almost identical effects, and side effects. This includes tolerance and the potential for complications in withdrawal, which is why I include them here and treat them the same as benzos in this book.

Some of the brand names of z-drugs are quite well known, such as Lunesta, Sonata, and Ambien.

And the thienodiazepines?

Thienodiazepines, like z-drugs, also have a very similar effect as benzodiazepines. They interact with the same receptor sites as benzos and as a result, have similar side effects. Bentazepam, brotizolam, clotiazepam, and etizolam are some of the common thienodiazepines. Some of their brand names include Clozan, Rize, Etilaam, and Pasaden. Just like z-drugs, I'll treat thienodiazepines the same as benzos throughout the rest of this book.

Is there a difference between the various benzodiazepines?

I mentioned potency, speed of effectiveness, half-life, and focus earlier. Now let's look at these in greater depth.

Potency - The original benzodiazepines, like Librium and Valium, differ significantly from the current drugs, such as Xanax, Ativan, and Klonopin, based on potency. This variance in potency can severely affect withdrawal.

Speed of Effectiveness - The speed of effectiveness can be broken down into two considerations: how quickly the drug takes effect and the duration of that effect. For example, diazepam (Valium) usually takes effect within 30–60 minutes and its duration can last days. Clonazepam (Klonopin) and alprazolam (Xanax) can take effect immediately while oxazepam (Serax) has a particularly slow onset. Clorazepate (Tranxene) and triazolam (Halcion) are short-acting agents lasting only 3–8 hours. The speed of effectiveness is important especially when benzos are taken for insomnia or when considerations need to be made for driving or operating heavy machinery.

Speed of Elimination (Half-Life) - Benzos also differ substantially based on how long the drugs take to become metabolized and eliminated from the body. This amount of time is measured by half-life, which is the amount of time it takes for half of the initial dose to be left in the blood. Some drugs like triazolam (Halcion) have a half-life of only two hours, while others like diazepam (Valium) can take anywhere from 20–100 hours to reduce to half of the initial dose. The speed of elimination often comes into question when people ask about long-term symptoms. Can the drugs stay in the system longer even if they're no longer found in the bloodstream, such as in brain tissue? This question is still to be determined.

Focus of Treatment - Some benzodiazepines focus on treating specific conditions more so than others. They even differ somewhat in their effects for more common conditions, such as anxiety and insomnia. Alprazolam (Xanax) and diazepam (Valium) are often used for treating anxiety disorders, while estazolam (ProSom) and triazolam (Halcion) are frequently taken for insomnia in addition to the z-drugs, such as eszopiclone (Lunesta), zaleplon (Sonata), and zolpidem (Ambien).

Are some benzos harder to withdraw from than others?

Some say that benzos are all the same when it comes to withdrawal and its symptoms. Others believe that it's harder to withdraw from the more potent benzos. Since much of the evidence is anecdotal at this point, it's difficult to make a scientific determination.

Ashton states in her manual that there is evidence that withdrawal from high-potency benzos can be particularly tricky.[87] The most potent benzos are alprazolam (Xanax), clonazepam (Klonopin), and triazolam (Halcion) and there is also some anecdotal evidence that the rate of protracted withdrawal is higher in those.

Still, there is one drug that seems to cause a more difficult and longer protracted state of withdrawal than all the others. That drug is clonazepam (Klonopin).

Now, I'll admit that my radar probably picks up more press about clonazepam than other benzos because it's the drug that I was on, so I might be biased. But I'm not the only one who has noticed this trend. And there might be some science behind it.

> *Clonazepam binds very tightly to GABA receptors, and this might be the cause of problems sometimes associated with withdrawal from this particular benzodiazepine.*[88]

— BenzoBuddies

There are so many factors including genetics, predisposition to addiction, environment, and others that affect the entire experience. In the end, any benzo can cause difficulty in withdrawal. Visit the "Types of Benzos" table in the appendix to see the detailed list.

The most critical factor is not the type of benzo you're on but the way in which you withdraw.

CHAPTER 3

EFFECTS OF BENZOS

Benefits of Benzos

Are there any benefits to benzos?

Of course, there are. I touched on this briefly in the benzo introduction, but let's take a deeper look here. Remember, the real question is not whether there are any benefits to benzos, but do the benefits outweigh the risks?

> *In my view, the only legitimate uses [of benzodiazepines] in psychiatry now are very short-term relief of catatonia, for severe agitation, and for detox from benzos. For everyone else, risk of addiction outweighs the potential benefit of use.*[89]

— Dr. Allen Frances, Professor Emeritus at Duke University

This is a hard subject to address fairly. This, in part, is because many people who have gone through benzo withdrawal feel that benzos are — for lack of a better word — poison. In their opinion, any benefits are heavily offset by the damage done to their bodies. That is the prevailing feeling in the benzo community, and I can relate.

> *...there is no place for benzodiazepines in the treatment of anxiety. There may be a place for them in anaesthesia, the management of*

epilepsy, or parenterally in states of acute psychiatric disturbance —
but that is all.[90]

— "A Policy on Benzodiazepines," 1987

Still, it would be nearly impossible for benzos to be so prolific if
they didn't provide some benefit.

Are there any benefits to long-term use?

Many people swear that benzodiazepines are wonderful. They love
them. Can't live without them. A lot of these people use them on a
short-term or as needed basis, but others swear by their long-term use
too. It's difficult to convince these folks otherwise. Since reducing the
dosage of benzodiazepines can cause difficult withdrawal symptoms
in long-term users, it's understandable that patients would be reticent
to undertake this action and even argue for a dosage increase. And I
don't blame them. Unfortunately, we're not always the best judges of
what is truly beneficial to our overall health.

While it might be a contentious topic in some circles, most government agencies and professional organizations now recommend
that benzos are prescribed for short-term use only, no longer than 2–
4 weeks.

Okay, then what are the short-term benefits?

In her speech, "Benzodiazepines: The Still Unfinished Story" from
November of 2000, Prof. Ashton stated that when benzos are used on
a short-term basis for insomnia, anxiety, seizures, surgical procedures,
and as muscle relaxants, they are rapidly effective, relatively safe, and
efficient.[91]

Still, even for short-term, these benefits do come with side effects.

How do benzos help with insomnia?

Benzodiazepines have a general hypnotic effect and can be quite
effective sleeping agents. That's the good news. Unfortunately, this
effect is usually short-lived. Most studies have agreed that long-term
use of benzodiazepines is similar to placebo for helping a patient

sleep.[92] A review by the *British Medical Journal* in 2013 concluded that people taking a sleeping tablet on a regular basis averaged just 25 minutes more rest a night.[93]

Benzos can be helpful with parasomnia, though. Parasomnia is a classification of sleep disorders that includes unwanted night time activity, such as REM sleep behavior disorder, sleepwalking, night terrors, teeth grinding, and others. Benzos, such as clonazepam, have been found quite useful in the treatment of some of these conditions.

How do benzos help with anxiety?

Benzos provide a generalized relaxed feeling and even a mild sense of euphoria in some patients. They help to calm down the brain and can quiet obsessive thought patterns that can cause extreme anxious episodes and panic attacks. The official guidance for use in treating anxiety from the Committee on Safety of Medicines (U.K.) advises that benzodiazepines "are indicated for the short-term relief (2–4 weeks only) of anxiety that is severe, disabling or causing unacceptable distress."[94]

Benzos have also been found to be useful in emergency room settings to calm extremely agitated patients or for psychiatric emergencies like acute psychosis, schizophrenia, or mania. Lorazepam and clonazepam are often used for these situations.

What about for seizures?

When benzos were initially released in the 1960s, they were prescribed for a variety of disorders including epilepsy. They are effective anticonvulsants and have been found helpful with seizures and as a muscle relaxant for muscle jerks.

For medical procedures?

The use of benzodiazepines in medical procedures is quite common and effective. Soon after benzos were invented, anesthetists were pleased to learn of their amnesic qualities, which allowed them to provide a premedication to patients that would help them forget difficult medical procedures or diagnoses. Think colonoscopy.

Midazolam is most frequently used in medical procedures since it's a strong sedative and provides fast recovery. Diazepam, temazepam, remimazolam, and lorazepam are also common.

As a muscle relaxant?

Benzos are strong muscle relaxants and have been found quite useful in treating painful muscle spasms. Tolerance does develop quite quickly, though.

Aren't benzos also used for alcohol withdrawal?

Yes. Benzodiazepines with a longer half-life, such as chlordiazepoxide and even diazepam, are often used to control agitations during alcohol withdrawal. It's ironic that benzodiazepines are used during alcohol withdrawal considering that the process of alcohol detox is quite similar to benzodiazepine withdrawal.

Adverse Effects During Use

And what about adverse effects, such as BWS?

If you don't mind, I want to hold on discussing benzodiazepine withdrawal syndrome (BWS) until Part II.

Okay, so are their side effects of benzos prior to withdrawal?

If you've ever read the complete list of possible side effects for a prescription medication, you will know that the list can seem endless. It can be almost like a mini-horror movie of possible aches, pains, conditions, and diseases. Well, the list for benzos is no different.

According to the Drug Enforcement Administration (DEA) in the U.S., adverse effects of benzodiazepines include aggression, antero-grade amnesia, delirium, depression, hallucinations, motor incoordination, paranoia, restlessness, and slurred speech.[95] Those are the highlights. Other sources add agitation, anxiety, blurred vision, confusion, constipation, difficulty breathing, dizziness, drowsiness, excitability, fatigue, headache, irritability, memory impairment, menstrual irregularities, muscle spasms, muscle weakness, sedation, sexual dysfunction, skin rashes, sleep disturbance, tremors, weakness, and weight gain.

Benzodiazepines may also aggravate other health conditions. According to the State of Pennsylvania Guidelines on Benzodiazepines, they can worsen the course of several conditions including chronic fatigue syndrome, depression, fibromyalgia, hypoxia (asthma, sleep apnea, COPD, CHF, etc.), and impulse control disorders.[96]

Still, as with any list of side effects, it's important to remember that this is a list of "possible" side effects only. No one will experience all the side effects above, and many of these are rare.

Can you die from benzos?

Unfortunately, yes.

There are two primary methods in which benzodiazepines are involved in mortality:

Overdose - Benzodiazepines are very common in overdose deaths, but rarely publicized since the more infamous players — like opioids — get all the press. In fact, some recent studies have even found that benzos kill more people than the illegal street drugs that we usually attribute to overdoses.

> *Benzodiazepines increase the risk of fatal overdose when taken in combination with opioid analgesics, alcohol, or other central nervous system depressants.[97]*

— New York City Department of Health and Mental Hygiene

As I mentioned in chapter two, the death rate from benzo overdoses exploded by more than 500% between 1996 and 2013, although this rate appeared to plateau after 2010.[98] Benzos are now involved in more than 30% of all overdose deaths.[99]

Detox - Benzos are one of the very few drugs that can actually kill you when you detox, similar to alcohol. Going cold turkey off benzos can cause severe psychological effects such as suicidal or homicidal ideation, psychosis, and hallucinations. In fact, both benzos and alcohol affect the GABA receptors in your body, and both can cause severe withdrawal symptoms, including seizures and even death.

And there appears to be a long-term effect on mortality as well.

...there is a 50% increase in overall mortality rates associated with long-term benzodiazepine use.[100]

— "Hypnotics' Association with Mortality or Cancer: A Matched Cohort Study," 2012

Should I drive while taking benzos?

A study published in 2000 estimated that benzodiazepines caused 1,600 traffic accidents and 110 driving-related deaths each year in the U.K. alone, and that number has most likely climbed since then.[101] According to *The Ashton Manual*, "studies from many countries have shown a significant association between the use of benzodiazepines and the risk of serious traffic accidents."[102]

You may have heard of this one: In May of 2017, Tiger Woods was found asleep behind the wheel of his car by the police in Jupiter, Florida. A police department video shows him slurring his speech while being interviewed. He was arrested under suspicion of driving under the influence, but his alcohol test came back negative.[103]

During the interview, Woods told the police officer that he had taken Xanax earlier that day. He was also on Vicodin, a prescription opioid, following back surgery in April of that same year. That drug combination can cause severe sedation and lack of coordination.[104] In fact, two weeks earlier Woods was filmed almost comatose in an embarrassing roadside video.

Benzos can affect driving or any activity that requires concentration and muscle coordination. They slow down the workings of your brain and muscles, which increases your risk of motor vehicle crashes. These side effects often ease over time, but since benzodiazepines should only be taken on a short-term basis, there shouldn't be an "over time."

A study in 1990 compared 4,554 people who had been prescribed benzodiazepines with 13,662 people who had been prescribed other drugs, but not benzos. The researchers stated, "We found accident-related care was more likely among persons who had been prescribed benzodiazepines." In fact, among those who had been prescribed benzos, "the probability of an accident-related medical encounter was higher during months in which a prescription for a benzodiazepine had recently been filled compared to other months."[105]

Benzos can affect your ability to drive safely. Please monitor your reactions closely before getting behind the wheel.

If benzos can cause amnesia for medical procedures, what do they do to everyday memory?

Cognitive dysfunction and memory impairment are quite common side effects of benzodiazepine use. Episodic memory (memory of recent events) is most commonly affected while some other memory functions may not be impaired at all.

Benzos can cause anterograde amnesia, which is the loss of the ability to create new memories after a specific event. So, if you take a short-acting benzo before a medical procedure, your ability to create a memory of that event is hindered, and you will have limited recollection of any uncomfortable events during the procedure. This is great for events such as an intrusive medical test, but not so great in everyday life. Whether this short-term cognition and memory issue gets better or worse in the long-term has been in debate, but some studies are starting to clear the muddy waters.

In 2004, a meta-analysis reviewed 13 small studies on benzodiazepines and found that long-term use was associated with moderate to severe adverse effects on all areas of cognition with impairment to IQ, information processing, visio-motor coordination, verbal learning and concentration, and most of all, visuospatial memory. The subjects in this study were all from withdrawal clinics so concurrent psychiatric issues and withdrawal complications might have limited its applicability.[106]

In the 1990s, the benzodiazepine triazolam (Halcion) was removed from the U.K. market. Allegations claimed that the drug caused severe psychiatric side effects including paranoia, hallucinations, and excitability.[107] Some patients have even claimed to have "black-out" episodes while on benzos. These are periods of time when the person has no recollection of what happened, or how he or she got there.

The effects among people suffering from PTSD, such as veterans, are particularly disturbing. PTSD is already a risk factor for developing dementia, and the use of benzos only makes it more complicated and, quite often, worse. In fact, the U.S. Department of Veteran's Affairs recommends against the use of benzodiazepines for the treatment of PTSD. Despite this recommendation, 30% of VA PTSD patients had a prescription for benzos in the fiscal year 2012.[108]

While the creation of memories about everyday life seems hindered by benzos, they appear to not affect semantic memory, language, or retrieval from long-term memory stores.

What about irritability, anger, and rage?

All of us get angry sometimes. When taking benzos, that irritability or impulse to lash out can be escalated and even worse, uncontrolled. The inhibitions that help us know the right course of action in certain situations are reduced, much like they are when we're drunk. When Halcion was taken off the market in Britain in the 1990s, one of the claims was that Halcion's side effects could be blamed for various criminal actions, including homicide. A Utah woman claimed that she murdered her mother under the influence of the drug.[109]

There are a collection of articles and studies that highlight the connection between benzos, anger, and aggression. I'll mention just a few short ones here, starting in the 1960s.

We have seen a number of previously quiet patients become assaultive and break up furniture in an office, shortly after being placed on chlordiazepoxide or another benzodiazepine, diazepam (Valium). In fact, even acts of violence such as murder have been attributed to the rage reaction induced by these drugs.[110]

— "Psychotropic Drugs and Induced Hostility," 1969

In the 1980s, Ashton elaborated on some of the concerns with a bit stronger language:

Patients may commit uncharacteristic antisocial acts such as shoplifting or sexual offences, or becoming aggressive with outbursts of rage and violence. Some researchers have suggested that chronic use of benzodiazepines may contribute to "baby-battering", "wife-beating" or "grandma-bashing."[111]

In 2014, a group of researchers in Australia performed a systematic review of benzos and aggression and found a "moderate association between some benzodiazepines and subsequent aggressive behavior in humans."[112] While attacks of rage and violent behavior have been reported in people with benzos since they were first invented, most of the time that irritability shows itself in much less threatening ways, such as anger and argumentativeness.

And what about depression?

People on benzos often suffer depression, especially with long-term use. Sometimes it's driven by their underlying condition, such as anxiety or insomnia, but many think that the benzos themselves contribute to depressive episodes in its users. This is especially true when it comes to emotional blunting.

I don't know that term. What is emotional blunting?

I can't help but think of Pink Floyd's classic, "Comfortably Numb," whenever I hear that term. Written by the great David Gilmour and Roger Waters, it truly captures the essence of emotional blunting, both musically and lyrically.

Hello? Is there anybody in there?
Just nod if you can hear me
Is there anyone at home?[113]

Emotional blunting, also known as emotional anesthesia, is quite simply the inability to feel pleasure or pain. It's like you have no emotions. Benzos are tranquilizers, and they sedate your emotional responses sometimes providing a general feeling of being numb.

Former long-term benzodiazepine users often bitterly regret their lack of emotional responses to family members — children and spouses or partners — during the period when they were taking the drug.[114]

— Prof. Ashton

Colin Moran, founder of *BenzoBuddies* (www.benzobuddies.org), one of the largest benzo support sites on the web, shared his experiences in an interview with ABC News. "I was a complete mess on benzos — confused, irrational, and unemotional." While on benzos, he decided to end his six-year romantic relationship. "It just felt wrong. When I told her it was over, she told me that the medication had changed me. I thought it was just a reaction to the breakup." After he was benzo-free, a flood of emotions overtook Moran. "I think it was just normal emotions, but it had been years since I experienced them and so, I wasn't used to coping with them," he said.[115]

I can relate to Colin's description. The inability to feel is a common complaint among benzo users. When I withdrew, the emotional landslide overwhelmed me. I still struggle to deal with many ordinary, everyday events. Benzos made me numb.

What about pregnancy?

Unfortunately, benzos and pregnancy don't mix well. Benzodiazepines are a class D teratogen. A teratogen is an agent that can cause a birth defect. A Class D teratogen is one in which positive evidence of fetal risk has been identified. Still, in some cases, the benefits may warrant continued use of the drug during pregnancy despite potential risks to the fetus.[116]

What are the risks to the unborn child?

Benzodiazepines taken during pregnancy cross the placental barrier and can affect the growth and development of the baby. These babies are more likely to be sick in the first few weeks of life and have their own withdrawal symptoms when they're born since the supply of benzos has been cut off. This is known as neonatal abstinence syndrome. These symptoms can include breathing problems, sucking difficulties, poor body temperature control, and poor muscle tone[117] — aka the "floppy infant syndrome."[118] Also, benzodiazepines are excreted in breast milk. NYC Health Info states that benzodiazepines should be avoided during pregnancy because of the risk of adverse outcomes for the newborn.[119]

It gets even more complicated for women who find themselves pregnant while already on a benzo long-term. Stopping cold turkey is not recommended, especially during pregnancy, but some say that a slow tapered withdrawal may be beneficial to the mother and newborn.

In "Guidance for Prescribing and Withdrawal of Benzodiazepines & Hypnotics in General Practice," NHS Grampian, a regional health board of NHS Scotland, advises the following:

> *Sudden cessation of benzodiazepine use during pregnancy is potentially hazardous for both mother and foetus, including the risk of convulsions. Benzodiazepines may cause long lasting and difficult-to-control withdrawal symptoms in the neonate, so any reduction in the level of use is to be encouraged.*[120]

Dr. Kimberly Yonkers studied the effects of about 2,600 women during pregnancy and after childbirth. Her study showed some risk from benzodiazepines including an increase in C-sections, reduction in the duration of pregnancy, and some infants needing respiratory support after birth. Still, Yonkers cautioned by saying "it should be reassuring that we're not seeing a huge magnitude of an effect here." Similar effects were also found with some antidepressants (SSRIs) in this study.[121]

Unfortunately, there are no easy answers here. Women should work closely with their doctor and decide what course of action is best.

Are children at risk?

Children have similar side effects and symptoms as adults and are not as equipped to handle the psychological and physiological changes triggered by these drugs.

At the annual meeting of the International Anesthesia Research Society in 2016, it was reported that a study performed at Vanderbilt University Medical Center found that "age, severity of illness and benzodiazepine exposure are the strongest predictors of delirium in critically ill children." Delirium is quite common in children with severe illness, and benzos have been found to only make it worse.

This is a poignant realization because currently the foundation of se-dation in the pediatric ICU setting is benzodiazepine administration. Understanding the relationship between benzodiazepine exposure with delirium and long-term cognitive outcomes in children is para-mount.[122]

— Dr. Heidi Smith, Pediatric Anesthesiologist

You mentioned Alzheimer's disease in a few studies. Are the elderly more at risk for complications from benzos?

If you meet an elderly patient who seems dopey, confused, has memory loss, slurred speech, and poor balance, your first thought should be benzo side effects — not Alzheimer's disease or demen-tia.[123]

— Dr. Allen Frances

According to the guidelines from the State of Pennsylvania, "extreme caution should be used prescribing benzodiazepines for the elderly, due to the increased risk of adverse reactions such as confusion, ataxia, and falls."[124]

Older people are more sensitive than younger people to the central nervous system depressant effects of benzodiazepines. Benzodiaze-pines can cause confusion, night wandering, amnesia, ataxia (loss of balance), hangover effects and "pseudodementia" (sometimes wrongly attributed to Alzheimer's disease) in the elderly and should be avoided wherever possible.[125]

— Prof. Ashton

One of the most pronounced dangers of benzo use in the elderly is the increased risk of hip fractures from falls. Old people fall. Old people on benzos fall more often.

A 2016 study from the University of Eastern Finland evaluated 70,718 people between 2005 and 2011. It found that benzodiazepines and related drugs increased the risk of hip fracture in patients both with and without Alzheimer's disease. In people with Alzheimer's disease, it increased the risk by 40%.[126] Quite often a fall is the start of a downward spiral of the person's overall health, which leads to disability and even death.[127]

Do benzos increase the risk of developing Alzheimer's disease?

I obsessed about this during withdrawal quite frequently. I'm good at obsessing. It's a gift.

A study released in 2014 by French and Canadian researchers linked benzodiazepine use to an increased risk of Alzheimer's disease. They found that the greater a person's cumulative dose of benzodiazepines, the higher his or her risk of Alzheimer's.

The researchers reviewed nearly 1,800 men and women over age 66 who had been diagnosed with Alzheimer's disease and compared them with a random sample of 7,200 others without Alzheimer's, matching for age and sex. They reviewed their prescriptions for at least five years preceding diagnosis. Those who had taken a benzo for three months or less had the same dementia risk as those who had never taken one. But, those who had taken the drug for three to six months raised the risk by 32%. And those who took it for six months or longer boosted it to 84%.

They also discovered that the type of drug mattered. Those who had taken a long-acting benzo — like diazepam (Valium) and flurazepam (Dalmane) — were at higher risk than those on a short-acting benzo — like triazolam (Halcion), lorazepam (Ativan), alprazolam (Xanax) and temazepam (Restoril).[128] In a 2016 analysis of eleven studies published concerning benzodiazepine use and the risk of dementia disorders, nine of these studies concluded these drugs have a harmful effect, one found a protective effect, and one (the most recently published) observed no effect. [129]

The researchers caution interpretation of these results stating, "The positive association found in some studies could be due to a reverse causation bias since the main indications for benzodiazepines (e.g., sleep disorders, anxiety) can also be prodromes [an early symptom] of dementia disorders."[130]

So, it appears that long-term use may increase your risk of developing Alzheimer's disease, but the studies are far from conclusive. Much more research needs to be done before any causal link can be established.

Is that it?

Unfortunately, no. There is also evidence that people who have
been on benzodiazepines long-term show a deterioration in personal
care and social interactions. Unfortunately, those most in need of support isolate themselves even further while on benzos.

Okay, now I'm done.

Tolerance, Dependence & Addiction

**I hear the terms addiction, dependence, and tolerance quite often.
Can you help me understand the difference?**

Sure. Let's start out with a few definitions from the National Institute on Drug Abuse (NIDA).

Addiction

*Addiction—or compulsive drug use despite harmful consequences—
is characterized by an inability to stop using a drug; failure to meet
work, social, or family obligations; and, sometimes (depending on
the drug), tolerance and withdrawal.*[131]

Dependence

*[Physical dependence is when] the body adapts to the drug, requiring
more of it to achieve a certain effect (tolerance) and eliciting drug-
specific physical or mental symptoms if drug use is abruptly ceased
(withdrawal).*[132]

Tolerance

*When drugs such as heroin are used repeatedly over time, tolerance
may develop. Tolerance occurs when the person no longer responds
to the drug in the way that person initially responded.*[133]

Dependence and addiction can be totally unrelated. One can be dependent and addicted, dependent and not addicted, or addicted and
not dependent. The NIDA clarifies this further by stating, "physical
dependence in and of itself does not constitute addiction, but it often
accompanies addiction."[134]

And as for tolerance, it means that your body responds less and less requiring more and more of the drug to get the same benefit. This can be tied with an increase in side effects and even symptoms like those experienced during withdrawal. This is called "relative withdrawal." Your body thinks it's withdrawing since it needs more and it's not getting more.

What is an addictive personality?

When I decided to withdraw, I told my doctor about my perceived "addiction" to benzos. He responded that I might be physically dependent, but he didn't think I was psychologically addicted. He explained that I did not have an addictive personality. I liked what I heard, but I wasn't entirely sure I understood. So, like everything else, I looked it up. What he was referring to as an addictive personality was a set of personality traits that may predispose me to addiction.

There is some controversy within the psychological community as to this topic, as there is with almost all topics. Still, there is a lot of evidence that supports the concept that someone with one addiction is more likely to develop other addictions than someone without any.

But, before I dig too deep into this topic of addiction, let's not. You probably know if you are drawn to addictions more than the next person. If you are, then withdrawal may be more difficult for you. If you are not, then things might be a bit simpler.

Unfortunately, propensity to addiction is only one factor that may determine your difficulty in withdrawal. One of probably a thousand. I was happy that I didn't have an addictive personality, but as I would later learn, that didn't mean that it was going to be easy. Not by a long shot.

So, can people be addicted to benzos?

Sure. People can be addicted to almost anything. Drugs, smoking, the Internet, cell phones, sex, bad relationships, trashy novels, gossip, cars, chocolate, picking lint out of your navel. You name it, we can all become addicted to something. Some people just have a higher propensity to it than others. By saying that benzos are addictive means that one can become psychologically addicted, physiologically dependent, or both.

But I'm not a drug addict.

Good for you. I'm not either.

I understand the gut reaction. Most of us who have been prescribed a drug by a doctor and wind up dependent feel betrayed. It's like we were secretly inducted into the drug addicts' world without our knowledge. Many in the benzo community are adamant about making a distinction here between dependence and addiction. It's important for them to differentiate themselves from addicts. But I try and look at it from a different perspective.

"Addict" is just a label. A label placed on a group of people who struggle with an addiction to a drug or drugs. Perhaps you picture someone in a grimy hallway shooting heroin. Perhaps you picture someone in and out of rehab five or six times. Rarely do we picture some college student at an Ivy League school who has taken a few too many Xanax. Especially when it was prescribed by a doctor without any warning.

According to most medical associations, addiction is a disease. Just like cancer, Alzheimer's, and heart disease. Some people are more prone to addiction than others. In fact, genetics play a huge role in determining who will be an addict and who won't.

I understand the desire to separate ourselves from drug addicts. The label is quite pervasive, and the connotation derogatory. If you were prescribed a benzo by your doctor, the desire to make it clear that you are dependent and not addicted might be quite strong. But whether we're dependent, addicted, or even dependent and addicted to benzodiazepines, we all need help. In fact, those who are addicted need even more help since they must struggle with their addiction in addition to their dependence. We're all in the same boat. No paddle. No radio. In the middle of a hurricane.

In this book, I try not to focus too much on labels. I'll use the term dependence more often than addiction since it's scientifically accurate for the subject matter. I'll also refer to the fact that many of us were prescribed this medication and had no idea what it was doing to us.

But please, if you're dealing with addiction too, don't feel ostracized. This book is for you just as much as it is anyone else.

So, when is drug use "drug abuse?"

Any drug can be abused, including benzos.

Prof. Malcolm Lader broke down benzo behavior in a way that makes sense to me. In his article "History of Benzodiazepine Dependence" published in the *Journal of Substance Abuse Treatment*, Prof. Lader categorized this topic into three main conditions and what behavior represents each:

> **Drug Abuse** - *Self-administration, large doses, outside medical context, drug-seeking behavior the rule*

> **Drug Misuse** - *Regular oral ingestion, large amounts, sometimes but not always obtained via prescription, typically starts within medical context*

> **Physical Dependence** - *Normal therapeutic doses, withdrawal syndrome of the sedative/alcohol type on discontinuation*[135]

What are the most addictive drugs? Are benzos on the list?

A 2014 article on *MentalHealthDaily.com* compiled a few studies to list the ten most addictive drugs. Here are the top ten in order of addiction rating,[136] starting with the most addictive:

1. Heroin
2. Cocaine/Crack Cocaine
3. Nicotine
4. Street Methadone
5. Crystal Meth
6. Barbiturates
7. Alcohol
8. Benzodiazepines
9. Amphetamines (Pure or Mixed Salts)
10. Buprenorphine

The first thing that came to mind when I looked through this list was that benzodiazepines are not in good company. The second thing

I noticed was that benzos were further down on the list than I expected. The truth is that while benzos might not be as addictive as
heroin, many medical professionals will tell you that withdrawal from
benzos is harder. This is mostly due to the drawn-out nature of
recovery, which can take months or even years.

Permanent Effects

**What about long-term or permanent effects? Do you ever worry
about that?**

Oh, yea. Plenty of times.

As far as long-term effects — well — it's a little late for me to start
worrying about that. I'm now four years off benzos, and I still have
symptoms. So yes, I'd call that long-term. As for permanent — well,
the jury is still out on this one. I don't want to scare anyone out there
who is afraid they might have permanent damage from the use of benzos — and that includes me. There is a lot of fear around permanent
effects, and I have willingly participated in that fear.

What does Ashton say?

Well, let's check in with *The Ashton Manual* on the subject:

*There is absolutely no evidence that benzodiazepines cause perma-
nent damage to the brain, nervous system or body.*[137]

— Prof. Ashton

Whew, that's done. That was easy. I love simple answers. Let's
move on.

**Wait a minute! So, you're saying that benzos don't cause permanent
damage?**

I was trying to provide the proverbial happy ending to the story
and move on quietly, but you're not going to let me do that, are you?
Unfortunately, that was not the only time that Ashton addressed this
topic. In March of 1995, Prof. Ashton said the following:

The question of whether prolonged benzodiazepine use can cause structural brain damage remains unanswered... It remains possible that subtle, perhaps reversible, structural changes may underlie the neuropsychological impairments shown in long-term benzodiazepine users.[138]

Are you good now?

What do other researchers say?

You really are quite persistent, aren't you? Okay, if you insist. Just remember, you asked. Let's travel back in time and see. Most of the research on brain damage with benzos was done in the 70s and 80s.

David Knott (1976) - As early as 1976, David Knott, a physician at the University of Tennessee said the following:

I am very convinced that Valium, Librium and other drugs of that class cause damage to the brain. I have seen damage to the cerebral cortex that I believe is due to the use of these drugs, and I am beginning to wonder if the damage is permanent.[139]

Malcolm Lader (1982) - Reported to the Medical Research Council on brain damage from benzodiazepines:

The results didn't surprise us because we already knew long-term alcohol use could cause permanent brain changes. There should have been a really good, large-scale study but I was never given the facilities or resources to do it.[140]

Isaac Marks (1989) - Marks, an anxiety specialist and colleague of Malcolm Lader, published a critique in the *Archives of General Psychiatry*.

The cerebral ventricular enlargement reported in patients with anxiety/panic disorders who were long-term benzodiazepine users could be due to the disorder or to other factors rather than to the drugs, but wisdom advises caution.[141]

Hans Bergman (1989) - Bergman and his colleagues did a five-year follow-up on sedative-hypnotics in patients who abused these drugs.

The results suggest that despite some neuropsychological improvement, cerebral disorder diagnosed in patients abusing sedatives or hypnotics is often permanent through the years and that neuropsy-chological status is linked to long-term prognosis.

This last study did involve patients who had abused the drugs so this may not carry over into the general population for therapeutic use. Still, it does raise concern about the possibility of permanent damage.

Sorry I asked. So, where does that leave us?

We now know a little more than we did in the 70s and 80s, but not a lot more. Studies appear to point to a causal link between benzos and dementia, including possible permanent brain damage, but they're far from definitive. The only sure thing that can come from this section is this: We need more research. And we need it soon.

Alternatives to Benzos

If I shouldn't use benzos, what can I do?

The good news is that there are quite a few alternatives. Yes, we all want the simple pill that will make our anxiety go away or help us sleep. Unfortunately, it's just not that easy. At least not without com-plications. Most of the alternatives take work or require a change in lifestyle. Still, there are proven methods that can work, and with some diligence, anyone can get better.

If you still want a pill, other medications can help, like SSRIs, SNRIs, melatonin, etc. But all these drugs come with their own set of possible complications. If you're like me and would like fewer pills, then there are many other non-pharmaceutical options. Or perhaps a combination is best. Only you and your doctor can decide.

Counseling and therapy have been the standard-bearer for psy-chiatric treatment of anxiety and insomnia for decades. Meditation and mindfulness are often integrated into these practices but can also be practiced on their own. Exercise is a tried and true friend and has been proven to be a consistently successful treatment option for a variety of conditions. Applied relaxation and exposure therapy are quite common techniques for treating anxiety. Assertiveness training has also been found to be beneficial. As for insomnia, several methods, such as autogenic training, progressive relaxation, feedback techniques, and sleep hygiene have been found to be quite beneficial.

Many of these techniques can be taught through a trained counselor or therapist, and a few of them can be tried on your own.

How effective is therapy, really?

Therapy has been proven to be a consistent form of treatment for anxiety, depression, and insomnia. Let's look at a study of Cognitive-Behavioral Therapy (CBT) and insomnia. According to Dr. Mark Porter in an article in *The Times*, "CBT has been shown to benefit three-quarters of people with insomnia significantly." He also suggests, "While you may not feel you can manage without your sleeping tablet, the latest research suggests otherwise." CBT has even been shown to help those who have been taking sleeping tablets for decades.[142]

In fact, the Veterans Administration and the U.S. Department of Defense recommend evidence-based psychotherapeutic interventions for their veterans with PTSD. A meta-analysis on the efficacy of treatments for PTSD published in the *Journal of Clinical Psychiatry* in 2013 suggests that psychotherapy is more effective than medications.[143]

I will talk a bit more about therapy later. Just know for now that therapy is a proven alternative to benzos as are other treatment options. There are alternatives. Some of them take some work, but it's worth it if you choose to be benzo-free.

CHAPTER 4

BENZO USAGE

Are benzos common as street drugs?

Yes, very. Many people don't even realize this. And they're especially lethal when combined with other drugs such as opioids and alcohol. As I mentioned earlier, benzodiazepines were involved in about 30% of all prescription drug overdose deaths in 2013, second only to opioids.

According to the U.S. Drug Enforcement Administration (DEA), there were an estimated 346,000 emergency department visits attributed to benzodiazepines in 2010. That's a 27% increase from 2008. In fact, according to the 2011 National Survey for Drug Use and Health, 20.4 million individuals aged 12 and older have misused benzodiazepines in their lifetime.[144] And the numbers continue to climb.

The National Center for Health Statistics (NCHS) and the U.S. Food and Drug Administration (FDA) examined federal data from death certificates between 2010 and 2014. They found that the most frequently mentioned drugs on death certificates in fatal drug overdoses included opioids, stimulants, and surprisingly, a class of prescription drugs called benzodiazepines. In fact, benzodiazepines made up two of the 10 most abused drugs on the death certificates. Those two benzos were alprazolam (Xanax) and diazepam (Valium).[145]

In 2016, the FDA issued a black box warning for the concurrent use of opioids and benzodiazepines. The black box warning is the strongest type of warning issued by the FDA and is required when there is reasonable evidence of serious or life-threatening risks associated with the drug, or in this case, a combination of drugs.

Why are benzos so dangerous in overdose?

> *If you mix a benzo with another drug that subdues your nervous system — painkillers, alcohol, antihistamines — the effects can be dangerous or deadly.*[146]

— Jennifer A. Reinhold, Philadelphia College of Pharmacy

Respiratory depression, also known as hypoventilation, is when breathing is too low or slow to provide adequate gas exchange, which increases the amount of carbon dioxide in the blood. It's the opposite of hyperventilation, in which you breathe too fast and get too much oxygen in the blood. As humans, we need a balance of oxygen and carbon dioxide, and when we get out of balance, bad things can happen. When benzos are combined with street drugs, such as cocaine, heroin, or others, this respiratory depression can become fatal.

As U.S. soldiers started returning from Iraq in 2008 with PTSD, some were dying in their sleep. Upon investigation, it was discovered that the cause was a cocktail of Paxil (antidepressant), Seroquel (antipsychotic), and Klonopin (benzodiazepine). This combination was routinely prescribed by VA hospitals.[147]

Most benzos are effective sedatives and muscle relaxants, which can be too effective when combined with other drugs. This combined effect can relax the body so much that breathing becomes too slow and too shallow. Due to this effect, benzos are contraindicated in people with obstructive sleep apnea, myasthenia gravis, bronchitis, COPD, and chronic pulmonary disease.

Mixing benzos with the following drugs can be dangerous: alcohol, antifungals, antihistamines (sedating), antipsychotics, barbiturates, cannabis, heroin, histamine-2 blockers, hydroxyzine, macrolides

(antibiotics), methadone, opioids, sleeping pills, and SSRIs.[148] The combined effect can lead to a variety of complications. In some cases, these complications can affect your thinking, motor functioning, and even breathing.

Where do people get these drugs?

The primary source of benzos is still doctors' prescriptions. But illegal acquisition is almost as easy. A simple Internet search can find a source within seconds. There is an underground market for benzos that appears to be quite lucrative for those who are involved in the illegal drug trade. That is until they're caught and go to prison. Then not so much.

So, what about benzos in the home?

As deadly as the benzo situation is on the street, the real "shadow epidemic" is in the home.

> *Much attention has been paid to the explosion of prescription opioid prescribing and the associated morbidity and mortality. Much less attention has been paid to the shadow epidemic of benzodiazepine prescribing and its consequences.*[149]

— Dr. Gary Reisfield, Professor of Psychiatry, University of Florida

The overprescribing of benzodiazepines by doctors, especially by general practitioners, is an epidemic. I'm not exaggerating this. I mentioned earlier that long-term benzo use in the U.K. and U.S. alone affects more than five million people. That is a huge number. It's more than the population of Chicago and Houston combined.

> *The culture in which we live sends messages that there is no reason to tolerate discomfort. That fuels misuse of prescription medications.*[150]

— Susan Foster, Vice-President and Director of Policy Research and Analysis, National Center on Addiction and Substance Abuse

The most frustrating part of all of this is that the warnings are there. From the government and even from the medical associations themselves, such as the American Medical Association (AMA), the American Psychiatric Association (APA), and United Kingdom's National Health Service (NHS). Still, doctors continue to prescribe them long-term.

> *[Benzos are now so mainstream that] psychiatric issues are sometimes being treated by primary-care physicians, who may not have enough training in or understanding of these drugs....people are in distress, and they want an instant cure—so it's hard for some physicians to withhold it, especially when they know they'll just get it elsewhere.[151]*

> — Dr. Stuart Gitlow, Addiction Psychiatrist and President of the American Society of Addiction Medicine

Many of the physicians have little training outside of their initial schooling, and the ongoing primary education is often being provided by the pharmaceutical representatives themselves. Most doctors honestly want to help their patients, and many of them still believe that these pills are doing just that.

> *When a patient comes in and tells you they can't sleep and want a sleeping medicine, there's a natural desire to try to please your patients. And it's so much easier to write the prescription than to have a long conversation about the risks and benefits of the sleep medication.[152]*

> — Dr. Kenneth Covinsky, Geriatrician at the University of California, San Francisco

Many of us are suffering from acute anxiety or insomnia. Many of us desperately want a solution. Something that will make us feel better. Something to take the edge off our daily crazy. We want some help, it's that simple. Unfortunately, there is no quick and easy solution.

In Aldous Huxley's dystopian novel *Brave New World,* the government distributed a pill called Soma. A happy pill. A pill that took the people away for a dream-like holiday within their own minds. Of course, in the story, this pill is actually a way for the state to control its citizens, to distract them from reality.[153]

Is it too late to say "spoiler alert?"

What is benzo usage like in the elderly?

Especially troubling is that benzo use is ridiculously high (nearly one out of ten) in the elderly, the group most likely to be harmed by them.[154]

— Dr. Allen Frances, Chairman of the DSM-IV Committee

Earlier, I reviewed some of the adverse effects of benzos in the elderly, which included a possible higher risk of developing Alzheimer's disease, general unsteadiness, hip fractures, and other various complications and side effects. Unfortunately, withdrawal is also more difficult for the elderly. An aging body loses its ability to restore itself over time in the way a youthful body does. Therefore, the return to normal functioning post-withdrawal can be more difficult and take more time.

In the United States, 8.7% of U.S. adults aged 65–80 were prescribed benzodiazepines over the course of a single year. This is despite the American Geriatrics Society (AGS) Beers Criteria, which includes a strong recommendation to avoid any type of benzodiazepine for the treatment of insomnia or agitation. The AGS also identified the use of benzodiazepines in older adults as one of 10 things physicians and patients should question.[155]

Just like with the rest of the population, overprescribing is the ongoing issue. A 2017 study in the *Journal of the American Geriatric Society* found an alarming number of older adults are being prescribed benzos without any diagnosis or alternatives even mentioned. In the study, only 16% of benzo users over the age of 65 had a mental health diagnosis, and less than 1% had been provided or referred to psychotherapy.[156]

Older adults have increased sensitivity to benzodiazepines and decreased metabolism of long-acting agents; in general, all benzodiazepines increase risk of cognitive impairment, delirium, falls, fractures, and motor vehicle crashes in older adults.[157]

— 2015 AGS Beers List

And what about the numbers for children?

According to IMS Health Vector One National database for the year 2013, over two million children under the age of 18 have taken benzodiazepines. As many as 700,000 of those are under the age of five. Since 2003, benzodiazepines prescribed for babies and toddlers has increased almost 300%.[158] There also appears to be an increase in violence amongst teens related to benzodiazepine usage over the past couple of decades.

According to the Johns Hopkins Psychiatry Guide, pediatric use should be limited. Safety has not been established for alprazolam (Xanax), clonazepam (Klonopin), or lorazepam (Ativan) in children. Only diazepam provides dosing advice for children under six years of age.[159]

CHAPTER 5

BENZOS IN THE MEDIA

Benzos in the Media? Getting a bit off topic, aren't we?

Well, maybe a bit. But I really like this chapter, so I'm keeping it in.

It's no surprise that a class of medication that has been around for over 50 years and has been prescribed millions of times has become part of the fabric of our society. It was inevitable. While the terms benzos, benzodiazepines, nonbenzodiazepines, or even z-drugs haven't necessarily entered the mainstream lingo as I mentioned in the introduction, brand names such as Xanax, Ativan, Valium, and Ambien have become ubiquitous in our culture. Since the media both influences and is influenced by almost every aspect of our everyday life, I believe it would be negligent not to talk about its effects here.

So, let's lighten the mood a bit and look at music, movies, and celebrities.

Okay. How about music? Can we start there?

Sure, why not? I know I mentioned this song earlier in the book, but I believe it deserves revisiting.

Mother needs something today to calm her down
And though she's not really ill, there's a little yellow pill
She goes running for the shelter of a mother's little helper
And it helps her on her way, gets her through her busy day[160]

— "Mother's Little Helper," The Rolling Stones

I remember this song well, although I'm sure that shows my age. No, I don't remember it when it first came out. I was only an infant at the time. But it became a classic, and as a classic rock fan, I enjoyed the Stones and their music. Still, I never really thought too much about the lyrics until recently.

The song first appeared on the Rolling Stones' album *Aftermath* in 1966. Most believe that the drug in question is Valium, although a few attribute it to Miltown. Many claim that it was a comparison of the drug-addicted life of a rocker with the drug-dependent life of a housewife. One approved by society, one not.

Either way, it was a commentary on the times. Valium was huge in the 60s, and it was a part of life. Pop culture, as it always has, comments on the trends of the day. Psychiatric prescription drug use, especially by women at home, was prevalent at the time.

"Mother's Little Helper" was not the end of benzos' reference in pop music. Here is just a sampling of some references through the ages; just for fun:

- 1972 - **Walk on the Wild Side** by Lou Reed – *"Then I guess she had to crash, Valium would have helped that bash."*[161]
- 1978 - **This Year's Girl** by Elvis Costello - *"Those disco synthesizers, those daily tranquilizers."*[162]
- 1988 - **Wild Wild West** by The Escape Club - *"Well, Mandy's in the backroom, handing out Valium."*[163]
- 1991 - **Big Mob on the Hill** by Leo Kottke - *"Concrete sheriffs, smiling, sighing, astroturf, benzodiazepine, Xanax, and gin."*[164]
- 2000 - **Lady Xanax** by Duran Duran - *"Oh, Lady Xanax where were you last night?"*[165]
- 2000 - **Feel Good Hit of the Summer** by Queens of the Stone Age - *"Nicotine, Valium, Vicodin, marijuana, ecstasy, and alcohol."*[166]

- 2003 - **Oxy Cotton** by Lil Wyte - *"Oxycontin, Xanax Bars, Percocet, and Lortab, Valiums, Morphine, patches, Extacy - and it's all up for grab."*[167]
- 2005 - **A Million Ways** by OK Go - *"Play that song again, Another couple Klonopin."*[168]
- 2007 - **I Feel Like Dying** by Lil Wayne - *"I am a prisoner, locked up behind Xanax bars."*[169]
- 2009 - **Something Is Squeezing My Skull** by Morrissey - *"Diazepam (that's Valium), Temazepam, Lithium...HRT...ECT, How long must I stay on this stuff?"*[170]
- 2009 - **Heartbreak Warfare** by John Mayer - *"Red wine and Ambien, you're taking shit again."*[171]
- 2009 - **Empire State of Mind** by Jay-Z, Alicia Keys - *"The city never sleeps, better slip you an Ambien."*[172]
- 2014 - **Klonopin** by Pill Friends - *"Tired of being awake, I'll take all your Klonopin...Won't be happy, won't be sad, but oh god it's for the best."*[173]
- 2015 - **Colors** by Halsey - *"Everything is blue, his pills, his hands, his jeans."*[174]
- 2016 - **Wildfire** by blink-182 - *"Living for the paycheck, dying for the weekend, take another Xanax."*[175]
- 2016 - **Two Birds, One Stone** by Drake - *"You stay xann'd and perk'd up so when reality set in, you don't gotta face it."*[176]
- 2018 - **Put Your Money on Me** by Arcade Fire - *"Above the chloroform sky, clouds made of Ambien."*[177]

Okay, I get the idea. What about TV and films?

The same. Benzos have shown up in popular TV shows and films since the early days of anti-anxiety medication. Valium and Xanax appear to get top billing here. Take a look:

- 1979 - MOVIE - **Starting Over** - Burt Reynold's character has a panic attack in Bloomingdale's department store. His brother shouts out, *"Does anyone have a Valium?"* Every woman in the store reaches in her purse and pulls out some pills.[178]

- 1999 - MOVIE - **Fight Club** - *"I've got a stomach full of Xanax. I took what was left of the bottle. It might have been too much."*[179]
- 2000 - MOVIE - **American Psycho** - *"She's usually operating on one or more psychiatric drugs; tonight I believe it's Xanax."*[180]
- 2002 - MOVIE - **28 Days Later** - Selena hands Jim some Valium to help him sleep. Jim responds, *"Oh, great, Valium. Not only will we be able to get to sleep, but if we're attacked in the middle of the night, we won't even care."*[181]
- 2002 - MOVIE - **The Hours** - *"I had this wonderful notion. I took the Xanax and the Ritalin together. It had never occurred to me!"*[182]
- 2007 - TV SHOW - **The Simpsons,** "Crook and Ladder" - *"I've read that people do strange things in their sleep when they've taken Ambien...I mean Nappien."*[183]
- 2008 - TV SHOW – **The Big Bang Theory,** "The Bad Fish Paradigm" - *"I gave him a glass of warm milk with a handful of my mom's Valium in it, but he still wouldn't shut up, so tag you're it!"*[184]
- 2010 - TV SHOW - **Fringe,** "Unearthed" - A doctor prescribes benzos for a teenager, and explains it to her mother, *"Benzodiazepine. It's a hypnotic, sedative, may cause a slight tingling sensation — it's actually quite pleasant. Besides, your daughter is 17. I'm sure she's sampled far worse by now."*[185]
- 2011 - MOVIE - **Bridesmaids** - *"No, you started it! Did you forget to take your Xanax this morning?"*[186]
- 2012 - MOVIE - **Silver Linings Playbook** - Tiffany and Pat sit at the dinner table sharing stories of their prescription drug therapies. *"Yeah, I was on Xanax and Effexor but I agree, I wasn't as sharp so I stopped." / "You ever take Klonopin?" / "Klonopin, yeah!" / "Right?!" / "Jesus!" / "What day is it?" / "Ha ha."*[187]
- 2017 - TALK SHOW - **The Late Show Starring Stephen Colbert,** "Colbert Mocks Trump" - Responding to some angry tweets from President Trump, Colbert comments: *"Who wakes that angry? Somebody get this guy a Xanax. Or a bran muffin. Or a bran muffin stuffed with Xanax. Like a Branax."*[188]

And that's just a very small sample. While the mention of benzos in the media can have an influence on its audience, I present these samples here more as a sign of the times and the pervasiveness of these drugs in our culture.

What about celebrity use of benzos?

The list of celebrities who have experienced the difficulties of benzos is long. Here are just a few which have drawn the public's eye: Tammy Faye Baker, Boris Becker, Chris Brown, Chris Cornell, Judy Garland, Margaux Hemingway, Paris Hilton, Whitney Houston, Choi Seung Hyun (T.O.P.), Michael Jackson, Heath Ledger, Courtney Love, John Mayer, Brittany Murphy, Stevie Nicks, Ozzy Osborne, Elvis Presley, Don Simpson, Anna Nicole Smith, Elizabeth Taylor, David Foster Wallace, Amy Winehouse...

Let's look at a few of these in depth for a bit more background.

Stevie Nicks - The lead singer of the 70s rock band Fleetwood Mac, Stevie Nicks, is perhaps the most well-known celebrity critic of benzodiazepine use. Nicks has battled addiction most of her life, including struggles with cocaine, heroin, and prescription drugs. When she was admitted to the Betty Ford clinic for rehab, she was introduced to clonazepam (Klonopin).

> *The only thing I would change is walking into that psychiatrists office who prescribed me Klonopin. That ruined my life for eight years. That's eight years that I could have. God knows, maybe I would have met someone, maybe I would have had a baby.*[189]

Nicks has described Klonopin as "a horrible, dangerous drug" and she added that it "turned me into a zombie." When speaking about her 47-day withdrawal from the drug she explained it as if "somebody opened up a door and pushed me into hell."[190] Nicks has since become a staunch critic of Klonopin and other benzodiazepines and speaks out at every opportunity to help prevent this horrible experience from happening to others.

I watched an interview with Nicks back in 2012 while I was in the middle of my benzo taper. I had just returned from the doctor's office feeling pretty good, but then I got sucked back into the Internet. I was craving some positive news, but when I came across the video, I couldn't turn it off. It was hard to watch, thinking to myself that what she went through is what I would go through. Still, I remember admiring her courage and resolve to stand up and warn others.

I am very grateful to Nicks for taking on this cause and being a cautionary example for those who follow. Thanks, Stevie.

Tiger Woods - I spoke a bit about Tiger Woods earlier in the book regarding his arrest while under the influence of benzos. Woods has been battling complications with his back for years and struggling with surgeries and medications. Unfortunately, mixing painkillers and benzos can have severe complications and can even be fatal. Hopefully, Woods has found a way to balance things out.

Chris Brown - Brown has become famous for his bad-boy attitude. In 2014, Brown was diagnosed with a mix of PTSD and bipolar II disorder, and he was reportedly self-medicating[191] with other drugs, including Xanax.

> *I was falling asleep on video sets. I was cussing people out randomly. I was doing crazy stuff. I would wake up, ask my homies, "Hey, man, so what time we gotta shoot this video?" And they'd be like, "Dude, we shot it yesterday."[192]*

Friends and employees have claimed that Brown is a sweet and sensitive guy, but his public reputation conflicts starkly with that assessment. Since irritability, aggression, and even violence are common side effects of chronic benzodiazepine use in addition to other drugs, it's possible that they may contribute to his behavior.

Luca Paolini - If you don't follow professional bike racing, you might not recognize his name. I must admit that I didn't. But in 2015, Paolini, a rider for the Italian national team, tested positive for cocaine while racing in the Tour de France. He said that he took the drug during training camp to help with an addiction to benzodiazepines.[193] He kept his addiction to benzos a secret, but eventually, he withdrew from the drugs with the help of his family. Paolini was banned from racing for 18 months.

John Mayer - John Mayer has said that he suffers from anxiety attacks and has feared that he would wind up in a mental institution.[194] He shared publicly that he keeps his anti-anxiety medication in his pocket at all times for his anxiety attacks.

Choi Seung Hyun (T.O.P.) - In 2017, K-Pop (Korean Pop) star T.O.P. had a life-threatening overdose and was rushed to the hospital in a near unconscious state. The Big Bang rapper was admitted to the hospital with severe respiratory depression and spent three days in intensive care.[195] His urine test later confirmed that he overdosed on benzodiazepines, which he took for anxiety. T.O.P. fully recovered and was released from the hospital. Unfortunately, that is not the case with many other celebrities on the list.

So, are you saying some celebrities have died?

Quite a few, actually. Here are some of the celebrities we've lost who struggled with benzos or had benzos in their bloodstream when they died:

Elvis Presley - On August 16th, 1977, Vernon Presley announced to the world, "My son is dead." The Los Angeles coroner's report stated that they found the tranquilizers Placidyl and Valium in his system along with morphine, Demerol, codeine, and an unknown barbiturate. [196]

Margaux Hemingway - In 1996, Margaux Hemingway, actress, model, and grand-daughter to the legendary author Ernest Hemingway was found dead in her Santa Monica apartment. She died of an overdose of barbiturates and benzos.[197]

Anna Nicole Smith - Smith was an actress and model who first garnered fame on the pages of *Playboy*. She is perhaps best known for her tumultuous marriage to oil tycoon J. Howard Marshall and the protracted legal battle following his death. Smith died on February 8th, 2007, at the age of 39. The investigation into her death stated that she died of an accidental overdose identified as combined drug intoxication. Smith had nine prescription drugs in her system, including chloral hydrate (a sedative) and three individual benzodiazepines, clonazepam (Klonopin), lorazepam (Ativan), and diazepam

(Valium).[198]

Heath Ledger - Known best perhaps by his role as The Joker in the movie, *The Dark Knight*, Heath Ledger's life was cut short at the age of 28 on January 22nd, 2008 before the film was even released. Ledger was found unconscious in his Manhattan apartment, and medical teams were unable to revive him. The medical examiner's report stated, "Mr. Heath Ledger died as the result of acute intoxication by the combined effects of oxycodone, hydrocodone, diazepam, temazepam, alprazolam, and doxylamine." Three of those are well-known benzos.[199]

Michael Jackson - Michael Jackson was perhaps the most famous pop singer of our time and was often dubbed, "The King of Pop." From the Jackson Five to *Thriller*, his songs topped the charts for decades. But in 2009, it all ended abruptly. On June 25th, Michael Jackson was found dead in his bed at his Los Angeles home. His death was ruled a homicide — involuntary manslaughter — by his own physician. The cause of death? The Los Angeles County coroner found the anesthetic Propofol in his body in addition to lorazepam (Ativan), midazolam, diazepam (Valium), and lidocaine. The physician's defense lawyer said that the singer swallowed enough lorazepam pills to put six people to sleep.[200]

Chris Cornell - The frontman for the band Soundgarden died on May 18th, 2017. He was found dead in his hotel room by apparent suicide. The night of his death, his wife, Vicky Cornell, spoke with him on the phone and said she noticed he was slurring his words, was acting different, and she was concerned he had taken too many Ativan.[201] She contacted security and asked them to check on him. His bodyguard found his body. A toxicology report noted that seven different drugs were found in his body, including a significant dose of the anti-anxiety drug lorazepam (Ativan), but the medical examiner's report said the drugs did not contribute to the cause of death.[202]

Tom Petty - Tom Petty, one of the icons of classic rock, was pronounced dead on October 2nd, 2017. He suffered drug toxicity from the mixture of benzodiazepines, an antidepressant, and opioids. Petty had been taking two benzos — temazepam and alprazolam — along with citalopram, oxycodone, and fentanyl. Petty was scheduled to have hip replacement surgery after performing on tour because he was under severe pain from a fractured hip. [203]

Lil Peep - Hip-hop artist, Lil Peep, was found dead on his tour bus in Arizona on November 15th, 2017, at the age of 21. The Pima County Office of the Medical Examiner noted that the cause of death was an accidental overdose due to the effects of fentanyl and alprazolam (Xanax).[204] The irony of the situation is that Lil Peep included his use of benzos in his music. In his song "Praying to the Sky," he wrote "I found some Xanax in my bed, I took that shit, went back to sleep. They gon' miss me when I'm dead."[205] Unfortunately, his lyrics were far too prophetic.

Well, so much for lightening the mood. There are plenty more, but perhaps it's best that move on to another subject.

CHAPTER 6

BENZO CREATORS AND REGULATORS

Benzos and Big Pharma

What is big pharma?

"Big pharma" is a nickname often used for large pharmaceutical corporations. The term has gained a negative connotation, almost to the level of conspiracy. And money is at the heart of it.

Now, I want to make it clear up front. I am not a conspiracy theorist, and I am not anti-drug. As I mentioned earlier, there are plenty of wonderful medications that save lives every day and wouldn't exist without the pharmaceutical industry. That is a fact. Many in the benzo community have become anti-medication — or at least anti-psych med — and I don't blame them. After what we have been through, it's easy to take that stance. And perhaps they're right. As for me, I try to be more objective with a middle-of-the-road mentality. I don't always succeed, but I try.

I don't have a problem with pharmaceutical companies. What I do have a problem with is some of the pharmaceutical company's practices. And that is what I will touch on here.

What is the size of the worldwide pharmaceutical market?

It's huge. In the year 2016, more than 810,000 people worked in the biopharmaceutical industry in the U.S. alone, generating $333 billion in total sales. That's $1,036 for each man, woman, and child. The total amount spent on healthcare in the U.S was over $3 trillion. [206]

Who is profiting from this business?

Well, if you want to make an enormous amount of money, be an executive at a U.S. healthcare company (which includes pharmaceutical companies). The highest paid U.S. corporate executives in 2016 were those within the healthcare industry. U.S. executives in health care averaged pay packages of $37 million per year, the most of any sector.[207]

What about drug advertising? I see a lot of drug commercials on TV. Has that increased?

I no longer watch the evening news. As many of you might relate, I turned it off because I couldn't handle the anxiety and negative thoughts it would generate. But I used to watch it every night. My wife and I would sit down at 5:30pm and turn on the nightly network news.

One of the things we noticed early on were the commercials. In my rough estimation, about 80% of the commercials during the nightly news were pharmaceutical ads. It was quite surprising. In fact, we used to notice when there was a non-pharmaceutical ad and wonder if the news had finished and we had moved on to *Wheel of Fortune*, which was often the case. The only exception to this rule was during a national election. That's when we wished the negative political ads would stop and we longed for the good old days of drug ads. How sad is that?

These ads you see on TV, they're what we call DTCPA.

What's DTCPA?

Glad you asked. See how I set you up there?

DTCPA stands for Direct-to-Consumer Pharmaceutical Advertising. Rules and regulations around this type of marketing have changed over time. Let's look at the history of pharmaceutical advertising in the U.S. to get a better understanding of how things have changed.

Since 1938, the Food and Drug Administration (FDA) has regulated the pharmaceutical industry in the U.S., which includes labeling and advertising. But little changed until 1981 when Merck ran the first direct-to-consumer print advertisement for a vaccine in *Reader's Digest* magazine. This was followed up in 1983 by Boots Pharmaceuticals when they ran the first broadcast ad promoting a prescription brand of ibuprofen.

The political landscape continued to change as the pharmaceutical companies put more pressure on the federal government to allow more marketing of their new drugs. In 1985, the FDA loosened the rules regarding DTCPA, which opened the flood-gates to enable print advertising. But broadcast was still limited due to the FDA's requirement that the advertisement must include complete information about all risks and side effects.

Then in 1995, the FDA loosened its regulations again. This time they required that the pharmaceutical companies only had to list "major risks" and provide an "adequate provision" that would direct viewers elsewhere to access complete information, like a phone number or website. Television ads inundated the airwaves. And then in 2004, the FDA loosened its regulations again.[208]

How much is spent on DTCPA?

Back in 1980, total spending in the U.S. on Direct-to-Consumer Pharmaceutical Advertising (DTCPA) was $12 million. Fifteen years later, the total was $340 million — an increase of almost 3,000%.[209] And it keeps growing. In 2016, total spending on DTCPA exceeded $6 billion.[210]

What other methods do they use to advertise?

On the front lines of pharmaceutical sales is the drug rep. These are the sales men and women who visit doctors in their offices to promote the latest drugs. In 2011, U.S. drug firms employed about 100,000 drug reps at the cost of $5 billion a year. Why did they do that? Because a successful rep campaign can bring in 10 dollars for every one dollar spent.[211]

But office visits are only part of the picture. Doctors are often invited to conferences at lavish resorts where they're offered a wide range of perks, including speaking fees, free gifts, and gourmet dinners.

Is there any attempt to increase regulations?

In 2008, Democrats in the U.S. House of Representatives tried to pass a bill banning TV ads during a drug's first three years on the market, but the billed failed to pass.[212] In 2015, the American Medical Association called for a ban on direct-to-consumer advertising stating that it inflates demand for more expensive drugs even when those drugs may not be appropriate.[213]

But it appears to be an uphill battle. Most of the efforts to stop DTCPA have stalled. The pressure from pharmaceutical companies and their lobbying bodies is overwhelming. In their defense, the companies claim that DTCPA is a free-speech argument and that the ads provide patients valuable information about treatment options.

What about benzos?

The number of people suffering from anxiety, insomnia, muscle spasms, and other similar conditions is probably around one hundred million in the U.S. alone. That's a lot of people. And that's also a very lucrative market for a drug manufacturer. Benzodiazepines accounted for nearly $509 million in sales in 2013 alone.[214] The drug manufacturers marketed benzos very effectively in world markets — enough so that Valium and Xanax became the best-selling drugs in the world in their respective time periods.

Still, most of the benzodiazepines are now off-patent, and the pharmaceutical companies that created them don't market them like they used to. The push from them has dramatically decreased.

Then where do the prescriptions come from?

I discussed some of the reasons in earlier chapters, including the fact that 90% of benzodiazepine prescriptions are prescribed by primary-care providers who may not have the proper training to diagnose and treat psychiatric conditions. Even though they're off-patent, benzos continue to be prescribed at a rapid rate.

Aren't you being unfair to these companies? Is there another side to the story?

There are always two sides. In an attempt to be fair and unbiased, let's take a look at the pharmaceutical companies' side of the argument.

First off, corporations are easy targets. Especially the big ones. They are run by CEOs, COOs, CFOS, boards of directors, and other extremely wealthy people. The vast wealth that this "1%" hold is more than many small countries. And this wealth quite often generates a bit of jealousy in the rest of us.

Big corporations are often seen as heartless, and that portrayal may not be entirely fair. Pop culture has helped elevate the modern corporate giant as the epitome of evil. Movies such as *Soylent Green, Wall-E, Jurassic Park, RoboCop, Ex Machina* and so many more have helped us question whether our corporate society benefits the individual person.[215]

And in the pharmaceutical arena, although many may dispute this, at least some of the blame lies with the patient. We want the quick fix. We want the magic pill. Drug companies are trying to give us what we ask for, and they spend millions in research and development trying to do that.

I share this information with you because I promised to try and be as objective and fair as I can be in this book. We need pharmaceutical companies. Medications have saved millions of lives, including mine, and someone must make them. We may want to paint the pharmaceutical companies as all evil, but it's never that simple.

Benzos and the Government

What about government regulation?

Most regulations are put in place to protect the consumer. When it comes to healthcare and pharmaceuticals, that means protecting the health of the patient. If large pharmaceutical companies were focused on safety first, then regulations would not be needed. But, when billions of dollars are involved, safety of the consumer often gets lost in the shuffle.

Nearly one-third of the drugs approved by the FDA from 2001 through 2010 had safety issues years after the medications were made widely available to patients. According to Dr. Joseph Ross, associate professor of medicine at Yale School of Medicine, of the 222 drugs approved, 71 were later withdrawn, required a black box warning (FDA's strictest warning) on side effects, or warranted a safety announcement about new risks.[216]

In the meantime, the federal government pushes for less regulation and faster approvals for new drugs.

Who governs the pharmaceutical industry?

This varies. Federal, regional, and local governments are the big players, but there are also medical associations and other regulatory bodies that have a say. And quite often, regulations in one area of the world can be completely different than in another, even though the risks and side effects of the drug are the same.

What are the current regulations for benzos?

Benzodiazepines are categorized as a Schedule IV controlled drug both in the U.S. and internationally, which means that the Drug Enforcement Administration (DEA) believes that they have a low potential for abuse and low risk of dependence. This leaves me as much bewildered as it does disheartened. The only exception to this is flunitrazepam, which is a Schedule III drug. The drug classification schedules rank current drugs based on the risk of abuse and harm. Here are the classifications from the DEA:

- **Schedule I** - High potential for abuse (no currently accepted medical uses) - Heroin, marijuana, Ecstasy
- **Schedule II** - High potential for abuse, with use potentially leading to severe psychological or physical dependence - Vicodin, cocaine, methamphetamine, oxycodone, fentanyl, Adderall, Ritalin
- **Schedule III** - Moderate to low potential for physical and psychological dependence - Codeine (90 mg or less), ketamine, anabolic steroids
- **Schedule IV** - Low potential for abuse and low risk of dependence - Benzodiazepines, z-drugs
- **Schedule V** - Lower potential for abuse than Schedule IV - Lomotil, Motefen, Lyrica, Parapectolin[217]

What is the regulatory situation in the U.K.?

Overall, the U.K. is well ahead of the U.S. and other countries in its concern about the dependency issues with benzodiazepines. There were warnings from the Department of Health (DOH) in 1980 and 1988 that benzodiazepines should be indicated for short-term use only.[218] This was followed in the early 1990s by the U.K. Committee on Safety of Medicines and the Royal College of Psychiatrists release of parallel guidelines. These guidelines restrict benzodiazepines to short-term use only, stress the need to establish a definite indication, and warn against abrupt withdrawal.[219] Unfortunately, it's still estimated that there are over one million long-term benzo users within the U.K.

In January of 2004, the Chief Medical Officer reminded doctors that benzodiazepines should only be prescribed for short-term treatment citing ongoing reports about problems with long-term use.[220] And the NHS Grampian, one of the regional health boards of Scotland, released its "Guidance for Prescribing and Withdrawal of Benzodiazepines & Hypnotics in General Practice" in October of 2006, which stated:

> *There are no licensed indications for the prescription of benzodiazepines for more than 2 to 4 weeks*[221]

In 2014, the National Institute for Health and Clinical Excellence (NICE) also warned that "benzodiazepines are associated with tolerance and dependence...therefore they shouldn't be used routinely to treat anxiety disorders."[222] And in Ireland, laws released in 2017 state that the sale or possession of benzodiazepines without a prescription is considered a crime under the Misuse of Drugs Act, much like heroin and cannabis.[223]

What about in the U.S.?

Unfortunately, the U.S. lags behind. I mentioned Senator Ted Kennedy's subcommittee hearing into the dangers of benzodiazepines back in 1979. Despite this legislative push by one of our most well-known senators, little was done on the federal level in the decades that followed.

The Food & Drug Administration (FDA) does recommend short-term use of benzodiazepines and warns that quitting benzos abruptly can result in severe side effects. In 2016, benzodiazepines also garnered a black box warning from the FDA cautioning patients and doctors that there are life-threatening risks of combining benzos with prescription opioids. The following year, the FDA expanded its warning focusing on three specific opioids: buprenorphine, buprenorphine-naloxone, and methadone.[224]

But unlike the U.K., little else has been done to publicize this underground epidemic on the U.S. federal level. That leaves some states and local municipalities to pick up the slack.

The State of Pennsylvania updated its "Prescribing Guidelines" from the State Department of Health on Oct. 25, 2016. This document warned doctors that benzodiazepines should not be the first choice to treat anxiety and should only be used for four to six weeks if needed. It encouraged doctors to get formal written agreements with their patients so that they have documentation that the patients are fully aware of the risks. The Pennsylvania guidelines also recommended extreme caution when prescribing benzos for the elderly or during pregnancy and lactation.[225]

In the state of Massachusetts, Representative Paul McMurtry has petitioned the State House on behalf of the benzo community. House Bill 3594 is titled, "An Act Relative to Benzodiazepines and Non-Benzodiazepine Hypnotics." The bill requires pharmacists to ensure that the prescription label includes a bolded, cautionary statement of the risks associated with long-term use and distribute a pamphlet created by the Department of Health that contains warnings about the medication. Also, the bill sets limits on refills and requires a patient's written informed consent.[226] The bill was filed on January 20, 2017, and as of May 2018, it's still without a vote in the House.

As I mentioned earlier in the book, the New York City Department of Health and Mental Hygiene published their City Health Information on "Judicious Prescribing of Benzodiazepines" in 2016. This contained some very strong warnings regarding the dangers of long-term benzodiazepine use.[227]

So, even though progress at the federal government level in the U.S. has been mostly non-existent, states and city governments are getting involved and picking up some of the slack.

Any progress in other countries?

Some countries have provided guidelines and regulations regarding the prescribing of benzos. Just for a sampling, let's look at Canada since they consume the second highest number of benzodiazepines in the world.

The College of Physicians & Surgeons of Alberta (CPSA) recommends the following:

Tolerance to the effects of benzodiazepines develops quickly (within weeks) and more of the drug is needed to achieve the same effect. Dependence can develop after only three to six weeks at prescribed doses.[228]

In 1992, Hong Kong regulated benzodiazepines under Schedule 1 of Hong Kong's Chapter 134 Dangerous Drugs Ordinance.[229] This forced doctors and pharmacists to keep detailed records of all benzo prescriptions. When comparing prescribing trends between 1991 and 1994, researchers found a 50% reduction in the average yearly number of benzodiazepine prescriptions per person.[230]

Still, the most progress is being made in the U.K. right now. Hopefully, the rest of the world will follow.

Are governments influenced by the drug lobbies?

Sure. All governments are influenced by lobbies, at least those that allow lobbying. This is the purpose of lobbying by special interest groups. Pharmaceutical companies are no different. The companies contribute to political campaigns and spend millions of dollars in lobbying efforts to influence laws that will benefit their industry. It doesn't seem fair to many of us on the sidelines, but this is how many governments work.

What about the APA and the DSM?

Now, I do not want to disparage the American Psychiatric Association (APA). I truly believe that the majority of their 47,000 members are well-meaning doctors trying to do the best for their patients. Still, the APA has come under fire at times for being too cozy with the pharmaceutical industry.

The common criticism is that members of the APA — just like the pharmaceutical companies — are driven more by income and profits and less by actual concern for their patients. Some even suggest that they use the DSM as a tool for generating this income. The DSM, or Diagnostic and Statistical Manual of Psychiatric Disorders, is the internationally recognized reference for classification of psychiatric disorders. The current version is the DSM-5, and some critics have questioned the politics behind the updates.

What happened in 2010 with Ativan and the MHRA?

You heard about that, did you?

In 2010, a group of cross-party members of the British Parliament pushed to increase funding into the dangers of benzodiazepines. Part of the reason for this push was caused by the issuing of 26 new generic licenses for lorazepam by the Medicines and Healthcare Products Regulatory Agency (MHRA). Why is this relevant? Let me explain.

Lorazepam was most commonly marketed as Ativan since 1972 by John Wyeth and Brother (Wyeth), who voluntarily canceled its license for "commercial reasons" in 2008. The MHRA, which is Britain's drug safety watchdog group, now issues licenses to pharmaceutical companies to manufacture and distribute the generic drug as lorazepam. When the 26 new licenses were issued in 2010, the new companies were to use the safety dossier and clinical trial evidence provided by the original manufacturer in their license application. But there was a snag: The safety information had been destroyed.

According to the law, the original manufacturer was not required to hold safety information beyond 15 years. So, Wyeth destroyed all the data. But that didn't stop anything. The MHRA issued new licenses to new companies without any safety information on the drug. Jim Dobbin, chair of the All-Party Parliamentary Group for Involuntary Tranquilliser Addiction, stated that the MHRA's policy of destroying drug safety information was "absolutely frightening" and "irresponsible."[231]

So, what does this all mean?

Okay, stepping on my soapbox for a moment here.

The playing field appears to be out of balance. Perhaps, at one point, the regulations were too strict and prevented growth. If that was once the case, the tide has now turned. Over the past few decades, pharmaceutical regulations have been stripped to the bare bones. Laws that protected the consumer by requiring stringent testing and maintenance of records have been gutted, and people like you and me are paying the price.

Life is about balance. The yin and the yang. We need balance. We don't need so much regulation so that it causes a parade of red tape and kills business creation, but we do need some laws so we're protected from pharmaceuticals that might harm us. Let's help encourage governments to create sensible regulations so that drugs like benzodiazepines can never do what they've done to so many people again.

Okay, stepping off the soapbox now. Thanks for listening.

CHAPTER 7

BENZOS AND THE LAW

What about lawsuits?

I don't want to spend too much time on litigation in this book, but it's difficult to cover benzo dependence without discussing it, at least briefly.

Litigation is a serious concern for both the pharmaceutical companies who manufacture benzodiazepines and the doctors who prescribe them. If physicians admit that benzos are addictive and dangerous, then they open themselves up to lawsuits from patients who have become dependent. And if pharmaceutical companies acknowledge that benzos are addictive and that long-term use can lead to ongoing or even permanent central nervous system damage, then they open themselves to massive class-action lawsuits, not only from individual patients but also from state-run health care programs.

Let's take a brief stroll through the litigation minefield and see where we stand today.

Is benzo litigation relatively new?

Not really. In fact, a class-action lawsuit against drug manufacturers was filed in the United Kingdom in the late 1980s involving 14,000 patients and 1,800 law firms. It alleged that the manufacturers knew of the dependence potential but intentionally withheld this information from doctors. This was the largest-ever class-action lawsuit against a drug manufacturer in U.K. history.[232]

The court case never reached a verdict. There were allegations that consulting psychiatrists had conflicts of interest and legal aid was withdrawn. In the end, the litigation led to changes in British law, making class action lawsuits more difficult to prove.

What about now?

More and more cases are being brought to trial, and many of them settle out of court for undisclosed amounts. Between 2010 and 2016, the Medical Defense Union in the U.K. paid out almost £750,000 in compensation and legal costs on behalf of members involved in 11 cases.[233]

Ray Nimmo, the founder of benzo.org.uk website, which houses *The Ashton Manual*, received £40,000 in an out-of-court settlement in 2002 after being prescribed Valium as a muscle relaxant for stomach pain in 1984.[234] Janet Waterton received £200,000 in a settlement from Devon Partnership NHS Trust after being prescribed benzos a second time when she had already been through detox.[235] And Luke Montagu, the Viscount Hinchingbrooke, suffered from benzo dependence for years after being prescribed them for a sinus infection. For 19 years he was prescribed a combination of drugs, including clonazepam. He received £1.35 million for his suffering.[236]

There are many more examples of previous and ongoing litigation regarding benzos, but I just wanted to touch on a few here.

Why are the lawsuits so hard to prove?

There are two key obstacles to litigation against the pharmaceutical industry. The first is money. Most plaintiffs can't compete financially with the legal teams paid by large pharmaceutical corporations. The second is the lack of studies and proof that benzos were the cause of the suffering that the plaintiffs claim. Despite all the warnings from medical associations and governments, it's still very difficult to get studies funded to prove that benzodiazepines are dangerous — especially when the pharmaceutical industry itself funds most drug research.

An article in *The Independent* by Nina Lakhani titled "Drugs Linked to Brain Damage 30 Years Ago,"[237] published in 2010, made some very serious claims as to how the U.K. government handled its funding of scientific research into benzos. In 1981, a group of government representatives and scientific experts gathered for a meeting hosted by the Medical Research Council (MRC). They reviewed research by Prof. Malcolm Lader that showed brain shrinkage in some patients of long-term benzodiazepine use, similar to that of long-term alcohol use. In 1982, the MRC agreed that large-scale studies into the impact of benzos were needed. Unfortunately, these studies were never carried out. In fact, the Department of Health has no record of the meeting.

Nina Lakhani claims *The Independent on Sunday* has seen the MRC documents and that they were marked "closed until 2014."

> *Many victims have lasting physical, cognitive and psychological problems even after they have withdrawn. We are seeking legal advice because we believe these documents are the bombshell they have been waiting for. The MRC must justify why there was no proper follow-up to Professor Lader's research, no safety committee, no study, nothing to further explore the results. We are talking about a huge scandal here.*[238]

— Jim Dobbin, Chairman of the All-Party Parliamentary Group for Involuntary Tranquilliser Addiction

Since 1982, the MRC has funded about 20 benzodiazepine studies, mostly with laboratory animals, but none of these followed up on the critical questions of brain damage. Prof. Lader had requested funding to follow up on his initial study, but the MRC denied his request.

How does this affect doctors?

There are a variety of ethical and legal dimensions when it comes to benzodiazepines for physicians. Is it ethical to prescribe benzos short-term? How about long-term? Is it ethical to withhold benzos from someone who requests them? Is it ethical to prescribe them for someone who is already on them and wants to withdraw? How about someone who is on them and doesn't want to withdraw? What about for a patient who appears to be drug-seeking?

It's not an easy position to be in. There are a lot of good doctors out there who only want to help their patients, and this litigation problem puts them in a difficult spot.

In the end, it's about money, isn't it?

Unfortunately, yes.

Both the pharmaceutical companies and physicians have a lot to lose if the litigation landslide starts to fall. The more we warn people about the dangers of benzos, the more interest there will be in legal action. These drugs are addictive, most government agencies and medical associations agree, so the word will get out and lawsuits will prevail. They already have in some areas. And once they do, the economic damage could be immense. The drug companies and physician groups know this and are trying to protect themselves in the meantime. Unfortunately, this means the patients are the ones left in the dark.

I sympathize with the doctors who are trying to do the best they can for their patients. But I also sympathize with the patients themselves, especially those who have suffered from benzodiazepine dependence. In my opinion, fear of litigation is not an acceptable excuse for millions to suffer.

Let's leave litigation now and take a look at incarceration.

What does jail have to do with benzodiazepines?

There's a story that I need to share here. It's a story that happened right here in my home state of Colorado. This is just one of many stories across the U.S., and perhaps around the world, that can and do happen when people addicted to benzos have to confront the justice system.

*** Trigger Warning ***

This next story may be disturbing to some. I am reporting it here because it needs to be told, but I recommend that you skip it if you're overly sensitive to the suffering of people in withdrawal.

When we dehumanize a group of people, any group, we strip away our sympathy for them. We start to care less and less until we feel that they no longer deserve fundamental human rights. We don't even blink an eye when atrocities befall them. John Patrick Walter was tortured to death. Yes, that's my opinion, and I know it sounds harsh, but after you read his story, you may understand my tone.

In April of 2014, Walter was arrested on charges of first-degree assault, felony menacing, and reckless endangerment[239] after getting into a fight with an acquaintance. He didn't have money for bail, so he was held in the Freemont County Jail until his arraignment when he would be formally charged. During his intake, Walter informed the staff that he was on some prescription medications,[240] which included 6 mg of Klonopin, a benzo. He even brought a list of his prescriptions with him.[241]

The U.S. Bureau of Prisons detoxification guide for "chemically dependent inmates" recognizes the dangers of benzodiazepine withdrawal.[242] And yet, Erik Heipt, attorney for Walker's family, claims that Freemont County had a "blanket policy" of not continuing benzodiazepine prescriptions for people in their jail,[243] therefore, forcing inmates to withdraw cold turkey. This is what happened to Walter. The following description of Walter's last days is summarized from an extensive interview that *Westword* had with Heipt.

In just 17 days in lockup, Walter lost 30 pounds. He exhibited delirium and exaggerated dramatic behavior caused by withdrawal psychosis and was often strapped in a restraint chair where he was tased and pepper-sprayed. When he was free of his restraints, he would kick and hurl himself against walls to the point of breaking bones. Other times he was disoriented, rolling on the floor yelling, and even seizing. Instead of receiving treatment for his withdrawal, John Patrick Walter received punishment.

For his final five days, Walter was placed in a holding cell with a large, see-through window for observation. As many as twenty people watched him at various times of the day. Everyone walking through the booking area could see him. While he was there, he didn't sleep or eat, and he drank very little water. And for most of the time, he was completely naked.

Many corrections officers were concerned and thought his medical providers weren't doing enough to help him. These complaints went all the way up to the sheriff, but in the end, they would always refer to the medical staff. A medical staff that just watched him deteriorate and never once took him to the hospital.

April 20th, Easter Sunday, Walter was on the floor naked twitching, shaking, and convulsing. That evening he was found dead.[244]

The cause of death was initially released as "undetermined." It wasn't until three years later, on April 17, 2017, that Dr. Emily Berry of the El Paso County Coroner's Office issued a revised finding. The official cause of death: "acute benzodiazepine withdrawal." Her revised statement was based on newly obtained medical records, eyewitness accounts, and materials furnished by the attorneys for Walter's estate, who filed suit in March of 2016.[245]

The medical staff who ignored Walter for 17 days worked for a for-profit contractor who was employed to provide medical services to its inmates. According to its contract with Freemont County, the company was paid $500,000 to provide medical services for the year of 2014, which is approximately $42,000 a month. And yet according to records, the company only budgeted $19,000 a month for on-site healthcare services.[246]

The Walter family believes that Freemont County tried to cover up what really happened during those three weeks.

> It goes to the core of our allegation that Fremont County engaged in a cover-up. That made it nearly impossible for the (coroner's office) to determine a cause of death. Now, through what's been uncovered, they have been able to determine a cause of death, which is what we suspected it was when we first filed this case.[247]

— Eric Heipt, Attorney for the Walter's Estate

I relate this story to you in my book for one reason — to raise awareness. The more people who know about benzodiazepine withdrawal and the dangers of withdrawing cold turkey, the less likely situations like this will happen. We need to educate the public and the medical professionals, so they're more aware of the dangers.

John Patrick Walter's death was preventable. If he had more money, he could have paid bail, and he would probably be alive today. If anyone at the jail had insisted he get help at any time over that three-week period, he would probably be alive today. If anyone on that medical staff truly understood benzodiazepine withdrawal, I believe, John Patrick Walter would probably be alive today.

What happened to Walter is inexcusable, and unfortunately, he is just one of many. The number of people who have suffered and even died from benzo complications and withdrawal while incarcerated is unknown. But here are a few examples to drive the message home.

Jesse Jacobs was jailed for 30 days on a DUI conviction in Texas. He died after just six days from Xanax withdrawal.[248] David Stojcevski died 17 days into his 32-day sentence in Michigan for a traffic fine. He lost 50 pounds, hallucinated, and experienced seizures and convulsions.[249] His death was caught on video, but the U.S. Attorney's Office found no evidence of criminal wrongdoing.[250] Cuyahoga County, Ohio has passed Sean's Law that protects people in jail who are on benzos.[251] It's named after R&B singer Sean Levert, who died in jail after being arrested for failing to pay child support. He arrived at jail with his bottle of Xanax in hand, but the drug was taken away from him, and he never received a single pill. The Cuyahoga County Coroner ruled that withdrawal from Xanax was a contributing factor to his death.[252]

I don't know about you, but I'm at a loss for words.

Let's move onto something else. Anything.

Good idea.

CHAPTER 8

OTHER BENZO STUFF

Benzos in the Economy & Environment

Tell me about the economic effects of benzos.

The socio-economic costs of long-term benzodiazepine use are un-quantified and perhaps unquantifiable.[253]

— Prof. Ashton

The economic damage of benzos is not limited to the individual. State-run health care programs and insurance companies cover a significant amount of the cost. This means that even if you don't take a benzo yourself, you're paying for them through taxes and insurance premiums. Other adverse economic effects include automobile accidents, increased sick days, cognitive dysfunction in the workplace, loss of productivity, unemployment, falls in the elderly, pre- and post-natal care for benzo-addicted newborns, legal costs, and incarceration from aggressive behavior and assault.

Prof. Ashton is right. The economic cost of benzos is unquantifiable.

You mentioned environment too. How is that a factor?

Here's an interesting one from the magazine *Science*. A study by Tomas Brodin and his colleagues at Umea University in Sweden examined perch, the freshwater fish, in the Eyris River in a densely populated region of Sweden. Now, you might wonder what fish have to do with this book. Well, hang on, I'm about to tell you. They found that these perch had concentrations of oxazepam in their muscle tissues. In fact, they had six times the concentration of the benzodiazepine than was in the water itself.[254] Similar levels of psych meds have been detected in water bodies near populated areas around the world. In 2017, ten species of fish in the Great Lakes region of North America were found to have high concentrations of Zoloft, Celexa, Prozac, and Sarafem in their brain tissue when examined after being caught.[255]

Where are they getting the drugs? Well, they're getting them from us. Mostly through our urine and into the wastewater. Benzos are now on a growing list of pharmaceutical products, including antibiotics, mood stabilizers, and sex hormones, that escape wastewater treatment facilities and get released into our freshwater sources.

This study raises at least two questions. First, how does this affect the fish? Is there enough concentration to have a physiological effect on these aquatic creatures? To find out, they exposed juvenile perch to varying levels of benzos. At concentrations twice the amount found in the Eyris River, the perch behaved differently. They were more adventurous, voracious, and more willing to explore. Basically, they were less anxious.

Second question. If these drugs are already starting to affect the fish in our rivers, are we re-ingesting the drugs through our drinking water? Officials point out that the concentrations of these pharmaceuticals are tiny and far below levels of a normal dose. They insist that our drinking water is safe. Still, the presence of so many over-the-counter and prescription medications in our drinking water should be a source for concern about the long-term implications. The U.S. federal government doesn't require testing for this and hasn't set any safety limits for drugs in water.

There's no doubt about it, pharmaceuticals are being detected in the environment and there is genuine concern that these compounds, in the small concentrations that they're at, could be causing impacts to human health or to aquatic organisms.[256]

— Mary Buzby, Director of Environmental Technology, Merck & Co. Inc.

Anything else?

No. Well, just one little thing.

One of the strongest benefits of benzodiazepines is their anxiolytic — or anti-anxiety — effect. They can be quite effective at helping us relax. They help us be more carefree. But can that go too far? For example, can benzos reduce our ability to feel empathy?

A study at the University of Chicago has investigated that. Results suggest that rats on benzos are less likely to help another rat in distress.[257] While some colleagues have questioned the actual interpretation of the results from this study, it still raises an interesting question. If benzos reduce our empathy for others, even a little bit, what does that do to our behavior when a family, friend, neighbor, or even a stranger is in need? Will we be less likely to respond? What might that do to a community as a whole? Will we be ruder to each other? Will we be more argumentative with each other? More irritable? Aggressive? Even divisive?

The Benzo Community

What do you mean when you say, "the Benzo Community?"

There's a community. An "underground" community might be the most accurate description. It consists of hundreds of thousands of people in all parts of the world. Patients. Caregivers. Even a growing number of medical professionals and scientists. It's a community of people who have had experiences with benzos either directly or through someone they know. This is the "benzo community."

Few of us have ever met one another, and yet, we rely on each other for support — sometimes life-saving support. Some benzo recovery groups have face-to-face meetings, but most of us gather on the Internet. Part of that is because it's effective in gathering people with similar issues together, but perhaps even more so because so many people who are suffering from benzo tolerance and withdrawal are reticent to even leave their houses, let alone meet with total strangers.

Either way, we're a community. And we're strong. We'll hang out on discussion boards and discuss our problems, ask questions, get advice, and gather the knowledge needed to survive this journey of withdrawal. Others of us have lived through withdrawal and stick around to help those who follow. Either way, it's a community of people helping other people in need.

So, you're a community. I get that. Do you have a leader?

There are leaders. There have been a lot of amazing and incredibly dedicated people working hard to help those in need. Some of them are medical professionals, some are politicians, some are community organizers, and even more of them are benzo survivors. All these people helped to build our benzo community. I, for one, am incredibly grateful to each one of them for the help and support they have provided.

Still, in the world of benzos, two names stand out above all the rest: Professor Malcolm Lader and Professor Heather Ashton. I have already referred to both multiple times in this book, so I think it's only fitting that I provide a little bit of background here about them.

Who is Malcolm Lader?

Professor Lader is seen by many as the original pioneer of research into the effects of benzodiazepine use and withdrawal. He is the one who first identified the so-called "benzo dependency syndrome" back in the 1970s. He even coined the term "opium of the masses" when referring to benzos. But most important, he sounded the first alarms about the destructive effects that benzodiazepines have on long-term users.

[It is] more difficult to withdraw from benzodiazepines than heroin.[258]

— Prof. Lader

What is his background?

Professor Lader is Emeritus Professor of Clinical Psychopharmacology at the Institute of Psychiatry, University of London, England, and a fellow at the Royal College of Psychiatrists. If you list Professor Lader's certifications it starts to look like an eye chart: Professor Malcolm Lader OBE, LLB, DSc, PhD, MD, FRC Psych, FMedSci. He has written 15 books and about 630 scientific articles on psychiatry and psychopharmacology. More than 100 of the articles were on benzodiazepines.

Lader has also held several distinguished posts including Adviser to the World Health Organization (WHO) on drugs in psychiatry, Adviser to the U.K. Ministries of Health, Agriculture, Defense and Transport, Honorary Fellow of the American College of Psychiatry, and President of the British Association for Psychopharmacology.

Prof. Lader has been campaigning for increased funding and research into benzodiazepine dependency for over 50 years. He has also tried endlessly to change prescribing guidelines and increase governmental warnings.[259] Unfortunately, this has been a long, lonely, and arduous battle.

What about Professor Ashton?

Many people in the benzo community will tell you that Prof. Ashton has helped more people withdraw from benzodiazepines than all the other people combined. And I would have to agree. Now retired, Chrystal Heather Ashton DM was a Fellow of the Royal College of Physicians, London (FRCP), a National Health Service Consultant in Clinical Psychopharmacology, a National Health Service Consultant in Psychiatry, and is Emeritus Professor of Clinical Psychopharmacology at the University of Newcastle upon Tyne, England.

Prof. Ashton worked at the University of Newcastle upon Tyne since 1965 as a researcher, clinician, lecturer, senior lecturer, reader, professor, and emeritus professor. She published approximately 250 papers in professional journals and books on psychotropic drugs and gave evidence to various government committees on tobacco smoking, cannabis, and benzodiazepines, and lectured on benzodiazepines in various countries.[260]

How vital is Prof. Ashton to the benzo community? Here's a perfect example. World Benzodiazepine Awareness Day (W-BAD) was founded on July 11th, 2016, to help raise awareness of the damage that benzos have done to the worldwide community. The date for W-BAD, July 11th, was chosen for a particular purpose:[261] It's Prof. Ashton's birthday. That's how important she is.

What is her specific experience with benzos?

In 1982, Professor Ashton established the first benzodiazepine withdrawal clinic within the British NHS and ran the clinic for 12 years. She studied the histories of over 300 patients and closely followed their progress.[262]

> For twelve years I ran a benzodiazepine withdrawal clinic for people wanting to come off their tranquillisers and sleeping pills. Much of what I know about this subject was taught to me by those brave and long-suffering men and women...It is interesting that the patients themselves, and not the medical profession, were the first to realise that long-term use of benzodiazepines can cause problems.[263]

— Prof. Ashton

When Professor Ashton closed her clinic in 1994 to retire, there was no one to take it over to continue her work. In 1995, she submitted a research proposal to the medical research council in the U.K. to "investigate the link between long-term benzodiazepine use and permanent brain damage." Her proposal was rejected.[264]

And what about *The Ashton Manual*?

In 2001, Prof. Ashton wrote a guide for benzodiazepine withdrawal titled *Benzodiazepines: How They Work and How to Withdraw*. It can be found today on the website benzo.org.uk, and it's free to anyone who needs it. This document is what is often referred to as *The*

Ashton Manual[265]

I have read over a thousand scientific studies, articles, websites, books, and other literature about benzos and related subjects during my withdrawal and in preparation for writing this book. Most of the ones on benzo withdrawal refer either directly or indirectly to *The Ashton Manual* at some point or another. Yes, when it comes to benzo withdrawal, all roads lead to Prof. Ashton.

But I don't want to read some droll scientific instruction manual. In fact, I'm even a bit scared of what it might say. Can't you just summarize it here for me?

I don't think that's a good idea. I will reference *The Ashton Manual* often in the coming chapters of this book, so, there will be some repetition. And that is by design. But if you assume that Prof. Ashton's writing is dull and too scientific — or even more so, too distressing — that is where you would be wrong.

The most surprising thing about her manual is that, despite the negative subject matter, it's quite uplifting. She is very optimistic that anyone, given the right information and planning, can withdraw from benzodiazepines. So, whether you read the rest of this book or not, please read *The Ashton Manual* before you withdraw.

You've also mentioned Dr. Frances several times? Who is he?

Allen Frances is a pre-eminent psychiatrist in the U.S. who is Professor Emeritus at Duke University and was the Chairman of the DSM-IV task force published in 1994.[266] He is also the founding editor of two well-respected trade journals — *The Journal of Personality Disorders* and *The Journal of Psychiatric Practice* — and is a contributing writer for *Psychology Today*[267]

The reason I add him here is based on an article he wrote that I came across in early 2017 titled "Yes, Benzos Are Bad for You." The article was initially posted on *Recovery Brands' Pro Talk/Pro Corner* in June 2016 and was reprinted on the *HuffPost* blog in July 2016, along with other sites.[268]

I was moved to tears when I read his article for the first time.

Finally, a current leader in the U.S. psychiatric community admitted in the mainstream media that benzodiazepines are addictive and that BWS is real. After all my research, this one article gave me the most hope for raising awareness in the U.S.

Why are you spending so much time listing the background of these people?

As I discussed in chapter nine, despite all the documented studies, government warnings, and expert testimony, there are still people who claim that benzodiazepine withdrawal syndrome is a myth or that our symptoms are just a re-emergence of pre-existing issues. So, to state my case, I believe it's important to detail the qualifications of those who back our claims.

Anybody Else?

Of course. There are thousands. The list of people around the world who have dedicated their time and money to help raise awareness, increase research and regulation, improve education, and support those people who are struggling is quite long. I'm afraid that if I start listing them here I'll omit someone inadvertently and I would hate to do that. So, for now, let's keep things simple.

Primary Goals for Change

Okay. You've covered benzos on the street, in the home, the elderly, the media, the government, the courts, the environment, you've discussed empathy and looked at the pharmaceutical companies themselves. You even extrapolated on your beloved "benzo community." With all of this going on, what can we do to change things?

Things are already changing. Unfortunately, it's been an excruciatingly slow process. As you may have noticed, I like to focus on positive efforts. I believe that real, lasting, beneficial change only comes from working with people, and not against them. So, I concentrate on five areas where I think we can make the most progress. These are awareness, research, regulation, education, and support. ARRES is how I remember it. It's a simple, silly acronym that works for me. If you'll indulge me, I'll briefly define each.

I don't have to be anywhere right now. So, what about awareness?

One of the first things so many of us are already doing is trying to raise public awareness. The more people who know about the dangers of benzos, the less likely they will start taking them. We need to change the narrative. We need to change the lexicon. Terms like "Xanax" and "Valium" are associated with relief and often the source of humorous dialog. It would be nice if those terms would instead have a more negative connotation, like heroin, cocaine, or even morphine.

What about research?

We need more research. We need to know more about benzos. What are the long-term effects? Permanent effects? Recommended withdrawal methodologies? We also need research into better treatment options for anxiety, insomnia, seizures, and muscle spasms. We need better, safer alternatives to benzos. We need funding for research so that we know the facts and stop guessing at the answers.

And regulation?

Many people in the benzo community are trying to increase support from the government, medical associations, watchdog groups, and any organization that has influence over the pharmaceutical and medical establishments. We need stronger safety regulations for the pharmaceutical industry. Reasonable regulations. Regulations that protect the patient. We need more studies and testing, and we need the government to help fund those. We need the governmental leaders whom we elect to start listening to us and help us deal directly with the problem.

What about education?

Educating patients and doctors on the facts about benzos is critical. Many doctors are still prescribing benzos long-term despite numerous governmental and regulatory agencies telling them not to. Doctors need to be reminded that there is no indication for a benzodiazepine prescription beyond four weeks.

We also need to make sure that they're educated on proper withdrawal techniques. No one should ever have to quit long-term benzo use cold turkey again. There is no medical need for this, and medical professionals need to know this. *The Ashton Manual* is free for everyone who wants to read it. We need to get it into the hands of more doctors, psychologists, pharmacists, and other healthcare workers. It shouldn't be left up to the patient to have to find out this information on his or her own, as so often is the case.

The College of Physicians and Surgeons in Newfoundland and Labrador in Canada along with Memorial University of Newfoundland have a great idea. They have developed a mandatory course for physicians on safe and appropriate prescribing practices for opioids, stimulants, and benzodiazepines. It's the first time that a college in Canada has mandated a course like this before new physicians can receive a license.[269] And I think it's a great start.

And finally, support?

The biggest of the five goals is support. There are thousands, perhaps millions out there who need help right now.

There are great websites and online communities, but we need more, and we need more people to know about them. We need more well-funded support groups and withdrawal clinics. Some of these clinics will need long-term residential accommodations, and that will be expensive.

Several support groups exist in Britain and are starting to pop up in other parts of the world. Still, most of these have little funding and are run by small charities. A 24-hour support line is also needed in most countries. This is a costly endeavor, but it can be a lifesaving tool for so many of those going through withdrawal. The British Medical Association (BMA) is on the right track. In 2016, the BMA said there needed to be more support for people with drug dependence and is calling for a 24-hour helpline.

Establishing a national helpline should be a top priority to provide better service to individuals with prescribed drug dependence...Patients have not had their problems adequately recognised in the past and we need to put that right.[270]

— Dr. Andrew Green, BMA's GP Clinical and Prescribing Policy Lead

We need more support from the government. We need more support from the medical community. We just need more support.

So, what can I do?

Talk with your governmental leaders and let them know that this is a major concern and encourage them to create and pass laws to help the pharmaceutical companies act more responsibly. That can make a huge difference. But there's another, even more direct method, that we can take in the short-term.

Ninety percent of the prescriptions for benzodiazepines come from general practitioners (GP) and not from psychiatrists. Some of these GPs prescribe benzos long-term because they don't know better, some because they don't believe the warnings they've read, and some probably because they only have seven minutes with each patient. One pill and the patient is happy — at least for a little while.

I am not anti-doctor. Far from it. I know that many of you have had some horrible experiences with your physicians or psychiatrists. I have too. But I've also had positive ones. I believe in my heart that most medical professionals have chosen their careers to help people. Some may have lost their way temporarily, but I still believe they are there to support and to help us heal. It may sound naive, but I know that we can change the system. And I believe we can do it one doctor at a time. I know this is possible because I've seen it happen, more than once.

While I was going through withdrawal, I saw a lot of medical professionals. Many of those professionals knew little about benzodiazepines and even fewer about BWS. I took the information I had researched, and I started my own little personal awareness campaign.

I presented my situation calmly and rationally (most of the time), and I backed it up by providing them with literature. Sometimes it was part of *The Ashton Manual*. Other times it was the article "Yes, Benzos are Bad for You" by Allen Frances. Those are two of my favorites. Doctors are skeptical by nature, so I made sure that the literature I provided was medically sound and from another physician with excellent credentials.

Over time, they saw my symptoms and my struggles. As they got to know me, they realized I was a rational person and that these "phantom symptoms" were not so "phantom." Some of them said they had other patients with similar problems and were connecting the dots. I'm sure many of them started to do their own research to check the validity of my claims.

Anyway, I kept doing this. And guess what? It made a difference. To this day I can count three medical professionals who have told me outright that they have changed their prescribing practices of benzodiazepines because I was their patient. I don't know about you, but I call that progress. Just think what would happen if every benzo patient could educate just one medical professional on the dangers of benzos and help them learn proper withdrawal procedures. What kind of difference could we make?

I believe that the biggest weapon we have in this fight against the overprescribing of benzos is us, the patients. One by one we're making a difference. It is happening.

Now let's look at withdrawal. What do ya say?

PART II
ALL ABOUT
WITHDRAWAL

Introduction

We're going to switch gears now. It's time to talk about benzo withdrawal.

Please keep this in mind: Part II is based on my personal experiences and research I have uncovered along the way. This is a conversation between the "old me" pre-withdrawal, and the "new me" benzo-free. Remember, everyone's experience is different. My experience won't be your experience. You should never substitute information in this book for professional medical advice. I am sharing these experiences with you so that perhaps some thought or story might make your journey go a bit easier. But these are only opinions and need to be treated as such.

In Part II, I will discuss all things in and around benzodiazepine withdrawal syndrome (BWS), including the symptoms, boundaries, difficulties, and some of the basics that I found to be useful for my withdrawal. Let's look at what's to come:

- **Truth and Controversy** - Is benzodiazepine withdrawal syndrome (BWS) real? The facts about this invisible syndrome.
- **What's It Really Like** - Personal stories of benzo withdrawal, including my own.
- **The Science of Withdrawal** - The science, the stages, and the taper.
- **The Symptoms** - The psychological and physiological symptoms of withdrawal.
- **Managing the Fear** - How to manage the number one enemy of a successful withdrawal.
- **Setting Boundaries** - Setting boundaries with food, drink, supplements, and other fun stuff.
- **The Natural Path** - Mindfulness, meditation, yoga, and spirituality.
- **For the Caregiver** - What's it like to be a caregiver to someone in benzo withdrawal and a few useful tips?

- **Benzo Free** - What's life like on the other side? When you're benzo-free?

Before we get in too deep, don't you want to remind me of the basics?

See? That's why we get along so well. We think alike. These may seem a bit repetitive, but just in case you skipped Part I or forgot some of the vital information, I think it's good to reiterate a few things here.

Taper Slowly, Under Doctor Supervision - If you choose to withdraw, then do so slowly in partnership with your doctor. Stopping benzos cold turkey, especially without medical supervision, can be very dangerous.

Remember, Everyone Is Different - This may not be a rule so much as an essential reminder. If you're anything like me, you may read hundreds of posts from people who have and are experiencing benzo withdrawal. As you do, keep telling yourself that everyone's experience is different. Most people post when they're at the most desperate point of their withdrawal, and therefore most of the postings are extreme examples. It's an unrealistic representation of the average withdrawal experience.

Use Common Sense - Everybody has opinions, and some of them can be quite strong. Use common sense, work with your doctor, and determine what is right for you.

Treat Suicidal Thoughts or Violent Ideology Seriously - Please, if you're having thoughts of a suicidal nature or of violence towards yourself or others, or if you know someone who is, seek help. Benzo withdrawal is a temporary situation. Life DOES GET BETTER! I am living proof of that. If you don't know who to turn to, I have listed several suicide resources in the appendix.

Okay, now back to the subject at hand...thanks for your patience.

CHAPTER 9

TRUTH AND CONTROVERSY

Okay, I'm just going to come out and say it. Is benzodiazepine withdrawal syndrome real?

Ah, playing devil's advocate, are we? I like it. In fact, I've been looking forward to this for a while. I'm ready if you're ready.

Good. So, how do you respond to people who doubt your illness?

First, let me provide a real short definition for the basis of this discussion. I'll elaborate more on this in chapter 11, but for now, let's keep it simple.

Benzodiazepine withdrawal syndrome (BWS) is the term given the collection of symptoms that occur in some people when they try to withdraw from long-term benzodiazepine use. These symptoms can last months and even years. For those of us who took benzos per a doctor's prescription, BWS is an iatrogenic illness — an illness caused by medical treatment.

Now that I cleared that up, I can honestly say that BWS is real. The symptoms that we experience are real. And, we're not alone.

Why should someone believe you?

I'm not saying they should. I wouldn't if I were in their shoes.

Hell, I've been where they are. I am a skeptic at heart. I had a friend who suffered from chronic fatigue syndrome. She complained about her disease and how bad things were. Our conversations were often negative, and at times, it was difficult to be around her. I even doubted the severity of her illness to the point of disbelieving it existed.

I'm not proud of those thoughts. She was a friend, and I should have believed her and offered to help her as best I could. Thankfully, my experience with benzos has increased my empathy towards those who suffer invisible illnesses. But, if you're asking if there are people out there who exaggerate or even make up an illness, sure, of course there are. But I believe those people are in the minority.

The truth is, I just want to get better. And most of us want the same thing. And if I could also help prevent this from happening to other people along the way, that would be awesome.

I've also heard some say that BWS is a scam, that it's an anti-doctor, anti-psychiatry cesspool of whiners?

Wow. That's a little strong, but I get where you're coming from.

Perhaps it does look like that on the surface to some people. I'll admit, some in the benzo community say that all medications are harmful. Or that psychiatry is a sham. Or that psych meds are designed to hook people until they die. And yes, there are a lot of angry people in the benzo community who have a gripe to bear. But, considering what they've gone through, can you blame them?

The only person I can speak for is me. We need pharmaceutical companies, medications, and especially doctors. I wish doctors were better educated on benzos and I'm not a big fan of some practices of pharmaceutical companies, but I don't believe that they're inherently evil. There's good and bad in almost everything in life, and these groups are no different.

I've also heard that BWS is a movement sponsored by Scientology to attack the psychological professions.

I've seen that too. Again, I can only speak for myself here. I can tell you right now that I am not a Scientologist. I really don't want to get into a religious discussion here, but I can honestly say that I have no ties to the Church of Scientology of any sort. In fact, I am a frequent patient of psychological counseling, and I believe that some psychiatric medications are beneficial. These are not, as I understand it, popular views within the Church of Scientology. So, I'm not sure we would agree.

What do you say to those who attack online support groups like *BenzoBuddies*?

All Internet groups suffer from problems. While they might provide useful information or help some people in need, they also have some members who are quite outspoken. The few more vocal ones garner most of the attention. I can tell you that most of the BWS online support groups that I have visited, including *BenzoBuddies*, have done a lot of good. They help people who are desperately in need find support, connection, and answers to their constant questions.

Those of us who suffer through BWS have a lot of symptoms. And these symptoms create a lot of questions. Unfortunately, outside of *The Ashton Manual*, there is not a lot of quality, medical literature out there readily available to us. So, we turn to benzo support groups. And they help.

And what about the ones who claim that BWS has 90 million symptoms?

It sounds a tiny bit high, doesn't it? I know the article you're referring to. I considered citing this article here so I could respond to its arguments directly, but the truth is, I don't want to add to its infamity. Is that a word? How about infamousnousity? Still no? Oh, it's infamy. Damn. I liked infamity better. I think it should be a word.

Anyway, this article argues that most of these groups support mass hysteria and wrongfully encourage people to stop medications that are helping them. It also contends that the list of symptoms that we claim is caused by benzodiazepine use is incredibly long. They use the 90 million number I hope as an exaggeration, but I get the point.

Now, the truth is, they're right — in a limited sense. It's true that some people on these boards do become influenced by repeated posts about the horrors of benzo withdrawal and some may develop psychosomatic illnesses. I'm sure that has happened. The brain is mighty, and it can create all kinds of effects based on confirmation bias. But you need to also consider this: Many people who come to these boards do so after they're already dealing with the difficulties of withdrawal. They didn't read about the symptoms first. Instead, they sought help because of their illness.

Throughout my withdrawal, I have had a variety of symptoms, and I'm sure that a few had absolutely nothing to do with my benzo withdrawal. The problem is that, during withdrawal, we don't know which is which. And that not knowing just adds to our anxiety and fears. Vicious cycle.

So, no, there are not 90 million symptoms. In fact, we have no idea how many there really are. It's too subjective. But, if someone asks me if there are a lot of symptoms for BWS — more than most illnesses — I would have to say yes. And I would have to say there is a good reason for it.

Long-term benzodiazepine use affects the central nervous system. So, it would make sense that symptoms of withdrawal, if they do exist, would be related to the central nervous system. Right? Here's the thing, though. The central nervous system, which includes the brain and spinal cord, is connected to everything. It's the thought processing and messaging highway for the entire body. So, if it is damaged, it would be logical that the parts of the body that it connects to might also be affected. That's a lot of possible symptoms.

So, is 90 million an exaggeration? Yes, absolutely. Is one hundred an exaggeration? Not so much.

> Thousands of people could not possibly invent the bizarre symptoms caused by the therapeutic use of benzodiazepines and reactions to their withdrawal. Many users have to cope, not only with a frightening range of symptoms, but also with the disbelief and hostility of their doctors and families. It is not uncommon for patients to be "struck off" if they continue to complain about withdrawal symp-

toms. Even when doctors are concerned and understanding about the problem, they often have little knowledge of withdrawal procedure, and even less about treatment...This is a drug-induced disease, not drug abuse.[271]

— Shirley Trickett, Journal of the Royal College of General Practitioners

And what about the people who say that they stopped taking benzos with no problem?

This is perhaps the most consistent argument heard from those who are skeptical about BWS. Some people stop taking benzos, even after long-term use, without any severe withdrawal symptoms. It's true. In fact, as I mentioned earlier, that number might be as high as 55%.

Some patients can withdraw from these drugs rapidly without great trouble. For others, it is a long, harrowing experience.[272]

— A. Byrne, Australian Family Physician

For now, just keep in mind that we're dealing with the central nervous system and it's complicated. And everyone is different. So just because one person had an easy withdrawal, it doesn't mean that the rest of us are making this up.

What about doctors who still say that long-term benzo use is not a problem?

The landscape is changing, but yes, there are a lot of medical professionals who still believe that long-term benzo use has few complications. This is one of the more significant frustrations for those of us in benzo withdrawal. If we can't go to our own doctor for reliable, accurate medical advice about the drug we have been taking, who do we turn to? You shouldn't attempt benzo withdrawal without medical supervision, so what do you do if your doctor doesn't believe you? I was lucky to find one who would work with me. For many others, that is not the case.

Some doctors appear resistant to believe that these drugs are addictive — a belief system that has existed for decades. In a 1976 study, researchers evaluated physicians' ratings of addiction for diazepam in two scenarios: one where the doctors knew it was diazepam, and the other where they didn't. Even though the researchers found "surprisingly strong evidence for diazepam's capacity to elicit tolerance and withdrawal," the physicians were less likely to accept that the drug was addictive when they knew it was diazepam.[273]

What's ironic is that most medical bodies and government health agencies don't recommend prescribing benzos beyond two to four weeks. And yet, doctors continue to prescribe them long-term and find it difficult to believe their patients who complain of related symptoms. Marion Brown, a psychotherapist working with the British Medical Association, describes it this way:

> There is a pattern in patients' notes where doctors don't believe that their withdrawal symptoms, such as pain, fits and psychiatric disorders such as panic and obsessiveness, are associated with the drugs... All too often doctors fail to take note of the fact they have been on benzodiazepines for years.[274]

This is all great, but I still don't see any evidence. Can you prove that benzodiazepine withdrawal syndrome really exists?

I was hoping you would ask that. Please bear with me for a little while. This is going to be fun.

First, here is Prof. Ashton referring to some research in the early 1980s:

> ...controlled trials demonstrated beyond doubt that withdrawal symptoms from regular therapeutic doses of benzodiazepines were real, and often severe, and that they indicated physical dependence on the drugs.[275]

Or perhaps a quick one from Prof. Lader:

> The benzodiazepines are now recognised as major drugs of abuse and addiction.[276]

I know, I'm already one step ahead of you. Prof. Ashton and Prof. Lader have been raising the alarm about benzo addiction for decades.

So, if you believe that they're part of the "benzo conspiracy," then I see how you might think they're tainted.

How about this?

Withdrawal from benzos can be more dangerous than withdrawal from heroin.[277]

— Dr. Stuart Gitlow, Addiction Psychiatrist and President of the American Society of Addiction Medicine

Not bad, right? Some of the strongest quotes come from Dr. Allen Frances, Professor Emeritus at Duke University:

The anxiety and panic experienced by people stopping benzos is usually much worse than the anxiety and panic that initially led to their use. Other common symptoms are irritability, insomnia, tremors, distractibility, sweating, and confusion. At the extreme, if doses were high and discontinuation is quick, the symptoms resemble alcoholic delirium tremens with hallucinations, psychosis, seizures, and the risk of death.[278]

How about this one from Dr. Jamie McAllister, a primary physician in Bend, Oregon?

They can have seizures, they can stop breathing. They can have hallucinations. It can be very scary. I've seen severe withdrawal from Klonopin, protracted withdrawal that lasts for months and months and months. All the benzos can be nasty.

She has a message to the other primary physicians who continue to prescribe benzos long-term to their patients:

So many times, I've wanted to call up the doc and say, 'Look, you started her on Klonopin, you take her off of it. You taper her and you walk through it with her and see what it's like. And I promise you, you'll never prescribe this s--- again.'[279]

Getting the picture?

Those are some strong opinions from individual doctors. But what about government and medical organizations?

I'm already one step ahead of you. In 2016, the New York City

Department of Health and Mental Hygiene published a City Health Information bulletin that stated this:

> *Facts: Benzodiazepine use can result in physical dependence at any dose with prolonged use.*[280]

That seems clear to me.

As early as 1980, the Department of Health in the U.K. warned that benzodiazepines are indicated for short-term use only.[281] In fact, in 2004, the Chief Medical Officer released a communication to all doctors stating:

> *Doctors are being reminded that benzodiazepines should only be prescribed for short-term treatment, in light of continued reports about problems with long-term use.*[282]

In 2006, the U.K. National Health Service / NHS Grampian made the following statements:

> *Benzodiazepines are potentially addictive drugs; physical and psychological dependence can develop within weeks of regular use.*

> *Dependence upon prescribed benzodiazepines is now recognized as a major clinical problem.*[283]

Sticking with the U.K., let's look at the British Medical Association (BMA). In July of 2016, the BMA stated the following in the documentary film *Benzodiazepine Medial Disaster* by Shane Kenny, former press secretary for Ireland's government:

> *Benzodiazepines can cause short and long term harm to patients when their prescription and withdrawal is not carefully managed. Not enough is known about the levels of dependence and withdrawal and the level of harm that is being caused. There is also too little research about the long term effects of these drugs.*[284]

Then, there is David Taylor, a spokesman for the Royal Pharmaceutical Society in Britain, who said that the society did not support the long-term use of benzodiazepines other than in "exceptional circumstances."[285]

Or one of my personal favorites from Anne Milton, Public Health Minister, United Kingdom:

> *I've met people who've been addicted to benzodiazepines for 20 or 30 years — wrecked their lives, wrecked their jobs, wrecked their families. It's a silent addiction. We all know about illegal drugs, we all know about alcohol, we don't know about this group.*[286]

Starting to think there's something to this?

Let's leave the U.K. and travel up to Scandinavia. Hafdan Pétursson is an Icelandic medical doctor and researcher for the Department of Public Health and General Practice in Norway. The following statement is from his research in the journal *Addiction*:

> *Physiological dependence on benzodiazepines is accompanied by a withdrawal syndrome which is typically characterized by sleep disturbance, irritability, increased tension and anxiety, panic attacks, hand tremor, sweating, difficulty in concentration, dry wretching and nausea, some weight loss, palpitations, headache, muscular pain and stiffness and a host of perceptual changes.*[287]

That sounds like the benzodiazepine withdrawal syndrome that we all know and love. How about if I pop back across the Atlantic to the U.S.? Here's one from Dr. Harris Stratyner, Vice Chairman of the National Council on Alcoholism and Drug Dependence (NCADD):

> *The two most dangerous drugs to detox off of are benzos and alcohol.*[288]

And finally, a few words from U.S. Senator Edward Kennedy back in 1979.

> *...these drugs [benzodiazepines] have produced a nightmare of dependence and addiction, both very difficult to treat and to recover from.*[289]

I get the picture. You can stop now.

As if I could. Don't give up so soon, we haven't even looked at the scientific evidence yet.

We actually knew from some experiments back in the 1960s that you could have dependence.[290]

— Prof. Lader

This dependence issue was initially assumed to exist only in high-dose users. In the 1970s though, studies started to focus on therapeutic-dose patients, and the results were alarming. Even people on doctor-prescribed doses were developing tolerance, and when they tried to withdraw, many patients found the experience just as severe as high-dose patients.

In 1979, The Institute of Medicine (IOM) at the National Academy of Sciences released its findings on sleeping pills. The following is from an article describing the panel's findings:

> *Sleeping pills, the most prescribed medication in the world, are more dangerous and less useful than either physicians or patients realize...the IOM report concludes that, although barbiturates are indeed as hazardous as everyone thinks, the chief alternatives, benzodiazepines, may be just as risky, and in some ways may be even more risky than barbiturates.[291]*

In 1983, a study was published in the *Journal of the American Medical Association (JAMA)* where benzodiazepine patients were switched to placebos at different intervals. Forty-three percent of patients who had been taking benzos for more than a year had withdrawal reactions. The number was only 5% for short-term users.[292]

Prof. Ashton's paper "Benzodiazepine Withdrawal: An Unfinished Story" published in 1984 methodically presents evidence based on her clinical experience working with patients who requested to withdraw from benzodiazepines. In that paper she summarized:

> *...these findings show very clearly that benzodiazepine withdrawal is a severe illness. The patients were usually frightened, often in intense pain, and genuinely prostrated. The severity and duration of the illness are easily underestimated by medical and nursing staff, who tend to dismiss the symptoms as "neurotic."[293]*

Still, there was a lot of doubt in the medical community. Many doctors claimed that the withdrawal symptoms were just a return of the original diagnosis. Others claimed that it was just hysteria. In 1990, a study published in *The Acta Psychiatrica Scandinavica* tackled the issue head-on. The study was titled, "The Prolonged Benzodiazepine Withdrawal Syndrome: Anxiety or Hysteria?" Is that on-the-nose or what?

The authors attempted to determine whether prolonged withdrawal symptoms were caused by the return of anxiety, hysteria, abnormal illness behavior, or the dependence process itself producing perhaps a prolonged neurotransmitter imbalance. It was concluded that the prolonged withdrawal symptoms were likely to be a genuine iatrogenic condition. Meaning, it was not caused by the return of anxiety, and it was not caused by hysteria. Its cause was likely a complication of long-term benzodiazepine treatment. [294]

In 1992, more evidence surfaced regarding flumazenil. I haven't talked much about this drug yet, but I will. For now, know that flumazenil is a benzodiazepine receptor antagonist. Sort of like a benzo antidote. It has been found in select studies to reverse some withdrawal symptomatology in patients. Unfortunately, it also has some severe complications. More on that later.

Anyway, this single-blind study found that intravenous infusion of flumazenil, and not saline, brought rapid relief of protracted symptoms including muscle tension, pins and needles, weakness, muscle cramps, jerks, burning, tremor, and shaking. These symptoms had been present in the subjects for up to 42 months from benzo withdrawal. The symptoms were improved by 27% all the way up to 82% in some.[295] The authors of the study stated that it was unlikely that the effects of the flumazenil were due to expectation, as previously assumed, because there was no response to saline injections.

I believe you. Please stop.

Okay, I'll stop. I guess I got a little carried away. I spent four years collecting that information, and I found it such a relief to know that I didn't imagine all my symptoms — that my illness was real. Thanks for bearing with me.

I'm convinced. But with all this evidence, why are they still being prescribed?

Ah, the billion-dollar question. We know the evidence is there. We know the warnings are there. And yet they're still prescribed long-term. What's going on?

> There's still a significant continuing problem with benzodiazepines in this country. We would have liked if it was solved 20 years ago, but it still exists...It's potentially a million people who are on drugs which only maybe is a tiny percentage of them need to be on, and that is not good for this country. It's also a waste of resource...We are ploughing money into these drugs and into support services for patients for a situation that we may have created ourselves.[296]

— Dr. Jim Kennedy, Royal College of General Practitioners

A 2017 study in *JAMA Psychiatry* uncovered serious over prescription and long-term use of tranquilizers despite concerns of the risks associated with long-term benzodiazepine use, especially in older patients. In fact, the study stated that more than 11 million people had prescriptions for benzodiazepines in 2008, and 31% of long-term users were 65 to 80 years old.[297]

There are a lot of groups fighting to change the laws and prescribing recommendations throughout the world, but it's an uphill battle in most areas.

> I came into this completely objectively, but the more I have delved into it, the odder the situation appears. I know all drugs have side-effects, but these are ruining people's lives... In my naivety, I thought the priority would be people's health. But if the priority is, in fact, a fear of litigation, then we have come to a pretty pass.[298]

— Eric Ollerenshaw, Tory MP for Lancaster and Fleetwood

Educating doctors on the dangers of benzodiazepine addiction and dependence is critical. There is a disconnect about benzos in the medical community, and as Eric Ollerenshaw said, it's "ruining people's lives."

CHAPTER 10

WHAT'S IT REALLY LIKE?

My Benzo Story

So, what's benzo withdrawal really like? Tell me your story.

Oh good, this is where I get to talk about myself. I wish I could say that I am too shy or humble to enjoy this, but I'm not.

I can tell. When did it all start for you?

I don't know the actual date when I was first prescribed a benzo. It was sometime in 2002. I was struggling with stomach issues. Pain, spasms, irritable bowel, heartburn. This was not new for me. I had my first upper-GI test at six-months-old and my first pre-ulcer condition at the age of five. Stomach issues were just something I lived with. We all have our burdens; that was one of mine.

I visited my primary care physician complaining about my stomach. We'll call him Dr. Y. I guess he thought he would try a different approach and prescribed an anti-anxiety drug to see if it might help my ongoing struggles. I have dealt with mild anxiety issues here and there, but it was never serious. I wasn't even complaining about anxiety to Dr. Y, but perhaps he thought it might be a factor.

Back then, I just trusted my doctor. I didn't question his judgment. So, I blindly took the medication. That drug was clonazepam (generic for Klonopin). I didn't know it was a benzodiazepine. I didn't even know what benzodiazepines were. There were no warnings. No mention of addiction or physical dependence. He said it might help my stomach, and that's all I knew.

How long did you take it?

I was on clonazepam for over twelve years. Eleven years on the medication and then tapered for a year and a half. I started at 0.5 mg daily and eventually upped my dosage to 2 mg daily in the last couple of years before tapering.

Were you in tolerance?

Yes, but I didn't know it at the time.

I had various symptoms that I now know are common with benzodiazepine tolerance. They were milder than what I experienced during withdrawal, so I either ignored them or got them checked out by the doc. I didn't think too much of it, and I never attributed the symptoms to the clonazepam.

I changed doctors occasionally during that time. Each time the new doctor would continue the prescription. In those first 11 years, not one doctor suggested that I should re-evaluate the medication I was taking. So, I kept taking the drug, naive to its effects on my mind and body.

When was the tipping point? When did you realize what was going on?

In the summer of 2012, I went to a new doc, Dr. G, for a physical. When I told her about the clonazepam I was taking, she said, without any alarm or apparent concern, that I should start to wean off that drug. This is the first doctor in eleven years to suggest that I shouldn't keep taking this medication. Still, I didn't think much of it. Dr. G first wanted me to get on an anti-depressant, so she prescribed me fluoxetine (Prozac), 40 mg daily. She said it would help me in coming off of the benzo. I wasn't too worried.

But then, a few nights later, my whole life changed in an instant.

I was trying to sleep on the twin bed in the front bedroom of our two-bedroom apartment. I had been snoring lately, so my wife and I were sleeping in separate rooms until I was able to lose some weight. I hated this, but it was the only reasonable decision since I kept waking her at night. This was my fourth day on Prozac, so I had just increased to my full dose of 40 mg that morning, per my doctor's instructions.

Anyway, sleep was evading me. I opened my iPad and decided to research Klonopin. I had nothing else to do, so I thought I'd kill some time. I can't believe that in the past 11 years I never researched this drug I was taking. A mistake I'll never make again.

It didn't take long for the panic attack to start. I came across horror story after horror story about benzodiazepine withdrawal. I was freaking out. In hindsight, I realize that this was my first, full-blown panic attack. I've had anxiety off and on in my life, but never something like this. I was terrified about what had been done to me and worse off, what was to come. I paced in my room for hours, and I knew that my life would never be the same.

I soon realized that my panic attack wasn't only caused by the fear of withdrawal, but also by an adverse reaction to Prozac. I've since learned that the prescription and dosage were inappropriate for someone in my condition. I stopped it the next morning just to be safe. Depression and a pervasive state of hopelessness set in soon after.

That was the start of my new journey. The withdrawal chapter of my life.

How long did your depression last?

I've been to psychologists a few different times throughout my life for depression. I was never diagnosed with any specific disorder, but I've struggled now and then. My first counseling session was in college after my girlfriend dumped me. For six months I was in a deep, dark hole and couldn't find any pleasure in life. I was never quite suicidal, but I could understand how people could consider it. It was an incredibly scary place to be and one I never wanted to visit again. Unfortunately, I wasn't that lucky.

I've never felt any stigma from visiting a therapist, so in the following years when I needed help, I'd find a local counselor and work through whatever the issues were at the time. Since this wasn't my first depression, I had a few tools and knew what to do. I started to build my team, my support system. I already had the most amazing wife in the world (no she didn't make me say that either), so now I just needed a few others to come along for the ride.

I found a new therapist nearby, and I started to journal, which I continued for the next five years throughout withdrawal. Since my memory was — and still is — somewhat rubbish, that journal became an integral part of the foundation for this book.

When did you decide to withdraw?

That first night. But I'd read enough to know that I needed help to do so. I didn't want to see Dr. G after the issue with Prozac. Instead, I mistakenly returned to Dr. Y, who originally prescribed the clonazepam many years earlier. No surprise that he told me to stay on the drug, that there was no danger of dependence. He even told me his wife had been on it for years. So, that wasn't going to work.

Still, I was steadfast in my decision to withdraw, and I tried again. I visited another previous doctor of mine, Dr. V. It was a three hour round trip to his office in the mountains, but it was worth a shot. I was comfortable with him, and I needed someone I could trust.

Dr. V is the idyllic small-town doc. He has a calming, wise presence and took his time each visit to listen to me, a quality that is difficult to find with today's trend of seven-minute appointments. He was the perfect fit for someone like me. We talked for over 30 minutes that first visit. I told him everything I had learned about benzos and about how freaked out I was regarding my addiction. He listened and discussed the issue with me at length.

Like most doctors at that time, Dr. V didn't believe there was a serious problem with long-term benzodiazepine use either. He said that I didn't need to withdraw if I didn't want to and that he had patients who had been on them much longer and at higher doses with no problems. Even though his words contradicted what I read over the past several weeks, and were quite similar to what Dr. Y said, I still felt that he was listening to me and wanted to work with me.

I told him that I didn't want to stay on the drug. I wanted off. And that after reading *The Ashton Manual*, I had a plan and I wanted to start immediately. He said he would work with me, but he wanted me to wait for six months before beginning my taper.

Six months? He made you wait six months before even starting to taper?

Exactly. And it sucked.

I hated that I had to wait. I believed that these drugs were destroying my body and mind from the inside and I wanted them out of me...now! I didn't want to wait one more week, let alone six months. I considered finding another doctor, but where?

A few days passed, and I calmed down a bit. I thought back on something Dr. V said in the appointment that — as hard as it was to admit — made some sense. He said he wanted me to stabilize mentally before starting my taper. I just wanted it all to be over.

Dr. V thought an anti-depressant might help, and after I shared with him my experience with fluoxetine (Prozac), he prescribed me a low dose of citalopram (Celexa). I took it as specified for the next couple of months, but eventually tapered off it before starting my clonazepam taper. I didn't have any adverse side effects from the SSRI, but I was determined to do this as medication-free as possible.

I realize now that Dr. V was walking a very fine line with me during that first appointment. I believe that he tailored his recommendations since I had heightened anxiety and first needed to address that issue. He didn't want to scare me with any more horror stories, and he knew quite well that if I started the taper in my current mental state, I probably wouldn't make it.

I am forever grateful to Dr. V for his wisdom, support, and especially his calm and compassionate manner. He was exactly the partner I needed for my withdrawal, and I am forever grateful.

So, did you stabilize?

The next month or two were hell. I couldn't stop obsessing about the benzos, what they were doing to my body, and what my future held. I was full of anxiety, and my depression wouldn't let go. I had some more panic attacks, lost work, and closed off from the world. I now realize that I was in tolerance at that time and already dealing with some withdrawal symptoms.

But, I did do a few things right. I started my sessions with a new psychologist. Celeste was great and incredibly supportive of my struggles. I also got a membership to a nearby gym and started working out and swimming again. It was during this time that I discovered yoga and meditation. Both have been vital to my recovery and to my life.

Over the following months, my tools slowly helped me to come to terms with my situation and stabilize my mood. I worked through some childhood and family issues with Celeste and developed some new tools to help with my anxiety. Finally, six months were up, I was more stable, and it was time to return to Dr. V.

How did it go?

It was February of 2013. I had my plan in hand. I had researched benzo withdrawal to excess, and I knew exactly what I needed to do. My mood improved, and I believed I was ready. Dr. V said he was impressed, and that he could see that my mental state had stabilized. I had taken charge and was in control of my own recovery.

He initially suggested a faster taper than I planned on, but I calmly told him that based on my research, a slower taper would be the best course of action for me. I suggested 0.25 mg every two weeks with the flexibility to stop and stabilize at any dosage for as long as needed. It was a little faster than recommended by Ashton, but I felt that it was appropriate for me at the time. I also decided to taper without the help of diazepam (Valium) as a substitution drug. The thought of adding another benzo to my system, regardless of its benefits, was more than I wanted to undertake.

He agreed to my plan and prescribed the proper dosages to start my taper. I was on my way. Yeah!

How did the taper go?

I wound up taking much longer than planned, and I'm glad I did. Over the next 18 months, I tapered off clonazepam on my own schedule. In the beginning, I didn't have many problems. But once I got down below one milligram (half of my original dose), my symptoms became stronger and I had more difficulty. It was a hard road.

Did you ever reinstate? Updose?

Unfortunately, yes.

In September of 2013, I started a new job at a marketing firm in Boulder. I was finally able to return to the business world, and I was hired to develop database systems for the company. It was exciting and terrifying at the same time.

My first day was hell. Filled with anxiety. Throat tightening. Tremors. Dizziness. Restlessness. My new office was a tiny half-cube in the middle of the hallway. I felt everyone was staring at me. My boss was in New York, and I didn't really have much guidance. Panic attack. Not my first, and not my last. I finally got through that first day, but I came home and told my wife that I didn't think I could do it. She listened, as she always does so well, and helped talk me down. Unfortunately, day one was a cake walk compared to day two.

The next day I had to fly to a convention in Baltimore. I know, crazy, huh? The anxiety was overwhelming. My physical symptoms were on fire. Shaking, spiders on my face, throat-tightening, muscle pains, tinnitus, etc. Flying never used to be a problem for me, but now my nerves were raw, and every little stressor was amplified. I almost canceled the trip multiple times, but it was a new job, and I knew I had to go through with it. No pressure, right? I hadn't traveled since I started withdrawal, and I was terrified.

In the weeks before the trip I had nightmares. I woke up in cold sweats wanting nothing more than to make the trip go away. But it had to be done. I forced myself to go to the airport and get on the plane and surprisingly, I made it through the flight. I meditated half of the way there. After I arrived in Baltimore, I checked in and went to the convention center and tried to fit in. But the worst wasn't over.

That night in my hotel I had another panic attack. And this was a bad one. I could hardly breathe, the world was spinning, I couldn't think straight, and I was all alone. What if something happened? Would anybody notice? What if my throat closed entirely and I couldn't breathe? What if my heart palpitations are a heart attack? What if? What if? I was pretty sure I was going to die.

I finally convinced myself, as so many of us do, that if I updosed just a little, it might help me get through. So, I did just that. I took another 0.25 mg going from 0.5 mg daily to 0.75 mg. It doesn't sound like much, but with such a potent benzo as clonazepam, it doesn't take much.

It helped for a little while. I made it through the rest of the trip and returned home. But the truth is, I probably would have made it through the trip without updosing. It just didn't feel like it at the time. It was six months before I started to taper down again. Updosing was a mistake, but we all make mistakes. I was in a challenging situation, and I did the best I could.

When did you jump (take your last dose)?

My last dose of clonazepam was on August 20, 2014. It was a great day, and I am so proud of that accomplishment. Unfortunately, it wasn't the end of the symptoms. In fact, it was barely the beginning.

What were your withdrawal symptoms?

Like most people going through benzo withdrawal, I suffered from a wide variety of symptoms that came and went through various stages of the process. This may look like a long list — and it is. Most people have far fewer symptoms than I did. Some of these symptoms were mild and periodic, but others were quite severe. Some of them lasted for only a few months, others, which I like to call my "greatest hits," have been with me for years. I'll go into more detail on these later but for now, here's a quick rundown:

- Akathisia (inner restlessness)
- Anger/Irritability
- Anxiety/Depression

- Benzo Belly (digestive issues, abdominal distention)
- Body Sensations (tingling, numbness, pain)
- Cognitive Issues/Memory Loss
- Dizziness/Vertigo
- Emotional Blunting (being emotionally numb)
- Facial Paresthesia (the sensation of spiders on my face)
- Flushing/Sweating
- Heart Palpitations
- Inflammation
- Insomnia
- Muscle Tics/Tremors/Shaking
- Muscle Tightness/Aches/Pain/Pulls/Tears
- Panic Attacks
- Pelvic Floor Dysfunction/Groin Pain/Abdominal Pain
- Personality Changes
- Restless Legs
- Sensory Hypersensitivity (nasal for me)
- Slurred Speech
- Throat Tightening
- Thrush (oral infection)
- Tinnitus (ringing in the ears)
- Urinary Issues

You weren't kidding. It's hard to believe you had all those symptoms.

I know. I even have trouble believing it, and I lived through it. But it happened, and it's still happening. I wish to hell it wasn't.

Do you think your symptoms are lasting longer than most others?

Yes, definitely.

I'm one of the 10–15% of long-term users who suffer from the protracted version of withdrawal. That puts me in the minority. My experience is extreme and is not a typical example of benzo withdrawal. Some have had symptoms 10 years or longer, but it's rare. Most withdrawal experiences will be shorter in duration than what I experienced, and that's excellent news.

Do you think your symptoms are more severe than others?

I know people who have tried to withdraw multiple times from a combination of drugs, including multiple benzos, and have yet to find success. I know people who haven't been able to leave their bedrooms for days due to overwhelming pain and anxiety. I know people who have had seizures, convulsions, and even temporary paralysis. I know people who have lost jobs, friends, and even marriages. And I am very sorry to say, I also know people who didn't make it and took their own lives.

It's tough to gauge the severity of my symptoms against others. Our experience of benzo withdrawal is incredibly subjective. But do some have it worse than me? Absolutely! Many have had it far worse than me. And it pains me every day to think about what they're going through.

What do you think caused your protracted state?

I have a few theories. I did make some mistakes during withdrawal. I tapered too quickly, especially toward the end. I updosed, which can cause problems. I also blindly took a specific antibiotic, which I later learned can aggravate withdrawal. And then there's the Klonopin factor. Most agree that those who take clonazepam (Klonopin) long-term have a higher incidence of protracted withdrawal than the other benzos.

Still, the real answer is that I have no idea. There are so many factors that can dictate what our withdrawal experience will be like, such as genetics, stress levels, mental stability, use duration, dosage, support systems, and diet. I may never know the real cause(s) of my extended symptoms, and that's okay. For now, I'm just focused on healing.

Did you work during your withdrawal?

Some. I worked on this book throughout my withdrawal when I had time. It helped keep me sane. I think the process of researching, logging, writing, and reaching out to people in the benzo community kept me centered and focused.

Before my taper, I was working as a contract screenwriter while teaching at college. I also helped organize and taught at various film festivals and conferences. I enjoyed working in the film industry and loved the writing and teaching. Unfortunately, my occasional writing contracts and adjunct college instructor salary didn't do a lot to support my family.

So, I returned to database work and got settled in the marketing firm in Boulder. I was moved out of the half-cube in the hallway and into my own private office, which helped significantly in managing my distractions and anxiety. The office where I was employed housed a division of the company that was focused on the natural food industry. So, I was surrounded by a lot of amazing people who were interested in eating and living a healthy life. I didn't know it when I started, but that was the perfect place for me to be at that time. They offered yoga, massage, a gym with a ping-pong table, and allowed me to bring my dog to work. I enjoyed the environment and especially the people I was privileged to work with.

I was tapering most of the time I was employed there. There were some hard times. Some real hard times. I tried to limit my sick days and worked from home on occasion as needed. I often traveled to corporate headquarters in NYC, which was very difficult at first, but over time I found ways to manage the stress. I converted my office into an anti-anxiety retreat with aromatherapy candles and soft lighting. I often worked through my lunches, but occasionally I would take this time to take a walk around the tree-lined streets, participate in a company-offered yoga class, or pop over to a nearby community center for some mid-day meditation. I buried myself in work which helped keep me focused. I did everything I could to mitigate my symptoms, and I believe I managed the situation quite well.

But when promised advancements continually got delayed, I started to get restless and began to return calls from the recruiters who were contacting me. Database skills were in high demand at the time. After 18 months at that company, I accepted a new job with a financial services company in downtown Denver, which almost doubled my salary. I traded an excellent work environment for more money. It felt like a no-brainer at the time.

I lasted four hours at the new job.

Four hours? Seriously?

This was not my proudest hour. I had a panic attack the first morning and quit before lunch. I have never done anything like that at a job before. On the bus ride home that morning, I just kept telling myself that this is not like me. What was going on?

It turns out that I had finished my taper and I was now in acute withdrawal. Tapering was a cake walk compared to this. My symptoms had kicked into overdrive. Plain and simple, I couldn't handle the stressors of ordinary, everyday life. And a new job, in a very stressful, open-office environment with co-workers staring at me all day long, was something my mind and body just couldn't handle.

I so badly wanted to return to my office oasis at the previous job where I could manage my symptoms in private. But that ship had sailed. I couldn't go back and ask for my job back. So, I went home, told my amazingly understanding wife that I was out-of-work, and started all over again.

Were you able to find another job?

Yes, for a while. I did database consulting for the next couple of years. I had two contracts with very prestigious companies, one for 12 months and the other for three. I was asked to extend both, but in the end, I had to leave each due to my health.

These failures at work really took a hit on my already struggling self-esteem. I knew that the main culprit in all these scenarios was my withdrawal, but that was little consolation when I couldn't provide for my family. Cognitive dysfunction, lack of short-term memory, and anxiety were the most significant problems at work. Oddly, I could still program in my core computer languages and develop database models in my sleep. Unfortunately, I couldn't learn new systems.

I still struggle with cognitive dysfunction today. It's like there's a wall. It's incredibly frustrating and just plain frightening. And as the pressure increases, the insomnia increases, and all my symptoms shift into overdrive. In fact, at my last contract position, I excused myself from work one morning in a state of panic with uncontrollable shaking. I was dizzy, nauseous, and almost in tears. I had to call to have my wife pick me up and drive me home because I wouldn't have been safe behind the wheel. That's not me. I've always excelled in my career. I've developed some of the top systems for some of the largest corporations in the country, but I just can't anymore. And that's a very bitter realization to accept.

So how are you doing now?

I was four years benzo-free in August 2018. Just saying that feels good.

Overall, I am doing well. Most days are good days, but I still have bad ones too. I struggle with my symptoms now and then and there are times that I let them get the better of me. Anxiety and cognitive issues are still a challenge, but I keep active and do my best to work around them. I also continue to have some insomnia, akathisia, tinnitus, paresthesia, and a few other mild symptoms, but I've learned to accept them, and they don't bother me as much anymore.

When I hit a wave, and my symptoms kick in, I remind myself of what it was like in the middle of withdrawal — on the worst of days — and remember how far I have come. I'm doing okay right now, and I know in my heart that I'm getting better every day.

Other People's Stories

What about others? What do they say about their experience with benzos?

I am just one in a vast sea of people suffering from this syndrome. And everyone's story is different. Here are a few personal accounts from others who have experienced benzo withdrawal and have shared their stories publicly.

*** TRIGGER WARNING ***

Many of these are extreme examples of benzodiazepine withdrawal. The horror stories. Please remember that withdrawal
from benzos is manageable. I am presenting these personal stories here to raise awareness and not to frighten.

*Benzodiazepine withdrawal should be called the Hypochondriac Dis-
ease. You will feel like you are dying and so many things are wrong
but most tests will show nothing is wrong with you, leading your doctors to believe you are crazy. I felt like I was having mini-seizures for
an entire month.*[299]

— Brooke Keefer, USA

*The "electric shock" waves became intensely painful and constant as
I reduced the Valium to zero at the end of 2008. A week after stopping, I had a terrifying fully conscious seizure that woke me up in the
middle of the night, practically paralysing me for three hours.*[300]

— Shane Kenny, UK, journalist and former Press Secretary for
the Irish Government

*I woke up and I thought I had a stroke, my scalp, down the middle of
my body — everywhere on the left was numb, and I could barely move
on that side of the body. Even though I thought I had a stroke, I was
in such a confused state that I didn't even feel inclined to do anything
about it.*[301]

— Colin Moran, USA, founder of *BenzoBuddies*

*The scariest thing is when you feel that you're going mad. I used to
think I should be in a mental home, I honestly did and I was really
scared, and I was thinking God, why am I like this?*[302]

— Suzanne Tovey, UK

*The last four years have been appalling, horrendous, hard work. I
would never live through that again. I would never wish anybody to
live through that. Yes, it's been awful. Really awful. I don't think she
[my daughter] will recall much of the last four years actually, being
on the tablets, because when I speak to her about it she says "I never
did that" and "I never did this." I said well you do Suzanne, you've
forgotten because you're on the tablets. Yes. So really she's lost those
four years in her life and she'll never get them back. So sad when
she's missed her teenage years.*[303]

— Pauline Whittam, Mother of Suzanne Tovey (above), UK

I didn't sleep for two months. I would be in fear states for maybe four, five, six hours a day. . . . It was almost like this primal feeling that you're about to be attacked by a lion; you're about to be killed.[304]

— Alison Page, USA

I have physical symptoms which are the palpitations, hot and cold sweats, shaking, trembling, to the psychological symptoms which is I think I'm going to lose it, I think I'm going crazy, I'm going mad — terrible pressure in my head.[305]

— Susan Hyatt, UK

My adult life has been destroyed by these drugs. Within two months of starting I made my first suicide attempt. I suddenly felt desperate and wanted a way out. I couldn't explain why my personality had changed so suddenly and dramatically. I would spend large chunks of the day asleep in bed and developed a fear of being alone. I was told that my symptoms were that of depression, and I believed it. I kept taking the tablets, thinking they would make me better. It never entered my head that it could be the drugs that were making me ill... I'm not a vengeful person; all I want is an acknowledgment that my symptoms have been caused by these drugs.[306]

— Fiona French, UK

Your Story

Okay, now I'm getting scared. I've been asking all these questions, but not sure I'm a fan of some of the answers.

I know. That's why I put the trigger warning in this section. It's human nature to read stories of other peoples' struggles and think their experiences are going to be yours. No matter what I say, reading things like that can be a setback for some people.

Benzo withdrawal can be hard. For some of us, it's the hardest experience of our lives. But for others, not so much. Proper management and preparation of your withdrawal can do a lot towards making this process easier. Thousands of people are withdrawing from benzos every day. You're not alone. You're not crazy. You can do this if you choose to.

But how do you know? You already said that my experience will be different than yours.

You're right. Perhaps you have been dealing with psychiatric issues your whole life and are sick and tired of trying every new drug and type of therapy when it comes along but to no avail. Or, perhaps you have never had a single psychiatric issue, but you were prescribed a benzo for muscle spasms from a sports injury and still can't fathom how you got here.

At the end of the day, it doesn't matter what your background is or what journey brought you here. You're hurting, and you need help. And you're reading this book, I hope, because you want to feel better. You want to get your life back. And you want to know what it's really like from someone who has been there.

I've been there. While your experience will most definitely be different than mine, many thoughts, fears, questions, and even some symptoms will be similar. I do know what it was like for me to go through benzo withdrawal and perhaps sharing my story and things I have learned will help you along the way.

You said you were scared during withdrawal. What were your biggest fears?

I had some mild fears and anxieties before benzos, as we all do, but during withdrawal those same fears became giants; and they were joined by some new and very powerful comrades.

Being overwhelmed is a common anxiety for me, and it grew to extremes during withdrawal, along with the new fear of being trapped. Of course, my old favorites, being abandoned and alone joined in. I also took my mild acrophobia to new heights — pun intended — which limited my travels and activities.

But my favorite fear during withdrawal is a real gem, and that is hypochondria. I've had so many symptoms during withdrawal, so many new pains, aches, and sensations, that it's easy to think something else is wrong. Something life-threatening. Something degenerative or disabling. I couldn't stop worrying. It's gotten better these past several months as I've found acceptance of my condition, but it's still there in the background.

Some nights I would even wake up choking, unable to catch my breath, and then stay awake for hours with fears of dying in my sleep. Or my chest pain would force me to contemplate another trip to the emergency room. I would also obsess that my benzo use will kick off early onset of Alzheimer's disease. My dad was diagnosed with Alzheimer's a few years ago, and since I still have cognitive and memory issues, this scenario haunts me even now.

So, what did you do?

I spent countless nights and mornings lying in bed worrying about my symptoms. It's what we anxious people do. My right brain hammering my left brain trying to convince it that I am dying of some illness. And my left brain calmly trying to rationalize saying that it's just the benzos — often with little effect. My mild, infrequent hypochondria that I had before withdrawal blossomed into full panic attacks during withdrawal. It was tons of fun.

Sometimes I went to the doctor and got checked out. In a one-year span, I had four EKGs, including some at the emergency room. I don't remember the number of doctors and specialists that I saw during my withdrawal. If I toss in physical therapists, massage therapists, acupuncturists, chiropractors, and others, it's probably over thirty different professionals with over a hundred separate appointments. I desperately wanted answers, and I would try anything that I thought might help.

Some nights I would sit and talk with my wife about my symptoms. She would calmly try and help me see the rational side of things. And it helped. Other times I would get on the online benzo boards and check my symptoms with others. It could be quite comforting to learn that others had the same issues I did and that it was related to the benzos, which it always was.

Eventually, I just had to resolve it in my head. Time would take care of that. Days would pass, and I didn't die. And my pain went away, or I got it checked out. Either way, I realized that it was just the benzos and I moved onto other things to worry about. Eventually, I found acceptance. But I'll talk more about that later.

What would you tell someone who is just starting out to help raise their spirits?

Well, here are a few of the thoughts that might help:

- Only about 45% of long-term benzodiazepine users will have a difficult withdrawal. And only 10–15% will have protracted withdrawal. The odds are in your favor.
- There a lot of things you can do to make withdrawal easier, including a slow taper, managing fear and anxiety, knowing your boundaries, and reducing stress.
- Thousands of people have gone before you and withdrawn from the drugs successfully, and there are a lot of resources to help you along the way.
- There is no hurry. In fact, slower is better. If you struggle at a specific dosage during your taper, you can stay there for a while and let your body adjust before taking the next step.
- There are a lot of other people going through benzo withdrawal online ready to talk at all hours of the day and night if needed.
- Doctors and the medical establishment are getting better at helping with withdrawal every day.

How do I know if I'll have a problematic withdrawal or not?

You don't. There have been no definite predispositions identified for benzodiazepine withdrawal syndrome. None that have clearly defined who will get it and who won't.

Think of it as a hurricane. As I'm writing this section, it's 2017, and Hurricane Harvey just finished its destruction of Houston and much of eastern Texas while Hurricane Irma is a couple of days away from Florida. A friend of ours has been staying with us from Houston for the past couple of weeks, so we have been watching a lot of the news coverage to keep up-to-date.

Anyway, think of preparing for withdrawal as if you were preparing for a hurricane. Stack up on water, food, gas, batteries, etc. Evacuate if requested. Do everything you can to survive the storm. And then, if it takes a sudden turn out into the Atlantic, you're good. No harm, no foul. Just an inconvenience. But if it does hit you head on, then you're ready. You're prepared. And you'll survive it better than most because of your preparation.

The same goes for benzo withdrawal. The more prepared we are, the better we fair.

> *With a sufficiently gradual and individualised tapering schedule...withdrawal can be quite tolerable, even easy, especially when the user understands the cause and nature of any symptoms that do arise and is therefore not afraid.*[307]

— Prof. Ashton

CHAPTER 11

THE SCIENCE OF WITHDRAWAL

The Science Behind BWS

How do you describe BWS to people who ask?

I have a simple description that I like to use in casual conversation when asked about my condition:

I have neurological damage caused by long-term use of a prescription medication.

While this definition may work well for friends and acquaintances, it does lack some of the details required for a more proper response. Upon my review of the literature on benzodiazepine withdrawal syndrome (BWS), the most concise and straightforward definition I found was on Wikipedia:

Benzodiazepine withdrawal syndrome—often abbreviated to benzo withdrawal—is the cluster of symptoms that emerge when a person who has taken benzodiazepines, either medically or recreationally, and has developed a physical dependence undergoes dosage reduction or discontinuation.[308]

What about protracted withdrawal syndrome (PWS)?

Protracted withdrawal syndrome (PWS) is a subset of BWS. BWS is often divided into stages including interdose, tolerance, taper, acute, and protracted. Protracted withdrawal just means that the symptoms have persisted longer than the acute phase, or longer than usual for most people who experience benzodiazepine withdrawal syndrome.

Why are benzos addictive? Why do people have difficulty withdrawing?

Any chronically used drug gradually engenders a series of homeostatic responses which tend to restore normal function despite the presence of the drug.[309]

— Prof. Ashton

Homeostasis is the human body's tendency toward physiological stability. When a new drug is introduced into your body, your physiology changes according to the effects of the drug. Eventually, through homeostasis, your body tends to re-balance itself — to find new stability. This process can often reduce the effects of the drug, which leads to the need for stronger doses. This is called tolerance.

As your body adapts to a benzodiazepine, it down-regulates the gamma-Aminobutyric acid (GABA) receptors, decreasing their sensitivity. So, GABA has less of an effect. And since GABA is an inhibitory neurotransmitter, the calming effect of GABA is less effective. The sensitivity of the glutamate receptors is also affected, but they become more susceptible to stimulation increasing the excitatory effect. The result is a decrease in calming influence and an increase in excitability. To learn more about GABA and glutamate, check out "The Science Behind Benzos" section in chapter two.

When a person discontinues taking benzodiazepines, all the physiological changes are exposed, which results in a rebound effect. The effect is generally the opposite of the initial effects of the drug. The homeostasis process kicks in again, but as before, this process takes time. Sometimes weeks, months, or even years. Eventually, stability is reached again, and the withdrawal symptoms subside. The body returns to normal.

After withdrawal, there also may exist what Ashton calls a learning deficit. While on benzos, the drugs aided in our psychological and physiological response to stress. We didn't have to develop — or learn — coping mechanisms to handle the anxiety. When the drug is removed, this learning deficit is exposed, and we have to create new synaptic pathways to manage the worries and complications of ordinary life.[310]

As I discussed earlier, there is also the possibility of structural neurological damage that may be long-term or even permanent in some people.

Are there other factors?

Sure. Earlier I talked about the effects of benzos on dopamine and its relation to addiction. Addiction studies have shown that benzos also affect the endocrine system. These studies have made it clear that the effects of benzodiazepines in the body are not limited just to the GABA receptors in the brain and central nervous system. Dopamine, CRF concentrations, and even hyperventilation syndrome might also play a part.

I have only listed a few studies here of the many that I have come across in my research. The science still has a way to go, but the good news is that we're gaining knowledge of how these drugs work and how they may affect a long-term user.

What are the odds of developing BWS?

This is another one of those debatable and somewhat controversial statistics. The answer depends on whom you ask.

The proportion of long term users of benzodiazepines in whom withdrawal symptoms may be expected to emerge has been variably estimated to be between 15% and 44%.[311]

— Study in The British Medical Journal, 1985

In general, a withdrawal syndrome is believed to occur in 30% to 45% of patients who have used regular therapeutic doses of benzodiazepines for more than a few months, but the incidence varies between less than 20% to 100% in different studies.[312]

— Prof. Ashton, 2011

I estimate about 20–30% of people who are on a benzodiazepine like diazepam have trouble coming off and of those about a third have very distressing symptoms.[313]

— Prof. Lader, 2011

Some 20–50% of BZD [benzodiazepine] users are believed to experience some sort of withdrawal when trying to discontinue BZD after extended use, indicating signs of dependence.[314]

— Study in *BMC Psychiatry*, 2015

...the incidence of withdrawal symptoms may be 100%.[315]

— Pétursson and Lader, 1981

It appears that the number is somewhere in the range of 15–100%. Is that specific enough for you?

Defining BWS can be complicated, and its inconsistencies may explain some of the variances in estimates. You first would have to establish benchmarks. How do you define "difficult withdrawal?" Is any withdrawal difficult? How do you define long-term? Eight weeks? Four? Two? You see the problem.

For the purposes of this book, I define long-term use as any regular, daily benzo use for longer than four weeks. And I define BWS, although it's still very subjective, as experiencing withdrawal complications including a cluster of psychological and physiological symptoms that can last for a few months to several years.

So, back to the initial question. I would say that approximately 45% of long-term benzodiazepine users will experience difficult withdrawal symptoms, or BWS. This is a composite number that I derived from various research, and I use it only as an estimate for the purposes of discussion.

What are the odds of developing protracted withdrawal?

Unfortunately, determining the percentage of long-term benzo-diazepine users who will wind up in a protracted state is just as diffi-cult to nail down. This is mostly due to different criteria as to when the protracted state of withdrawal starts.

In earlier studies, researchers defined the acute phase of with-drawal as lasting only one month and anything past that time would be protracted. Since then, we have learned more about the actual length that this syndrome might last, and with that new understand-ing, the time frame has expanded accordingly. Drawbacks in earlier studies included limited time for evaluation. They didn't stay with the patients long enough to see how they were doing after months or even years.

Most numbers for protracted withdrawal syndrome hover around 10–15%, but those were often based on the protracted phase starting at anywhere from one to six months.[316] Here's an example:

For some chronic benzodiazepine users, withdrawal can be a long, drawn-out process. A sizable minority, perhaps 10% to 15% develop a post-withdrawal syndrome, which may linger for months or even years.[317]

— Prof. Ashton, 1995

In this study, Ashton defines acute withdrawal as lasting 5–28 days, so the protracted phase would start after only one month with-out benzos. It would make sense that if we extended the acute phase to last multiple months, then the percentage of those still in with-drawal in the protracted state would drop. In fact, some sources have stated that it's as low as 3–5%. But not all agree.

Surveys have shown that about 15–30% of the patients continue to report significant symptoms from 10 months to 3.5 years following the withdrawal of these drugs.[318]

— Afzal Javed, Journal of Pakistan Medical Association

This article looks at protracted rates over a more extended period and still shows a similar percentage of people with long-lasting symp-toms. Which, like so many questions about benzos, leaves us without a definite answer.

For the purposes of this book, I have decided to stick with Ashton's original number (10–15%), which appears to be the consensus.

> *It is estimated that 10–15 percent of people who took benzodiaze- pines long-term (past the 2–4 week prescribing guidelines) will ex- perience protracted withdrawal or a 'post-withdrawal syndrome.'*[319]

> — W-BAD Website

What determines who will have to go through BWS?

We don't really know. As I mentioned earlier, there has been no clear predisposition identified. Some say that duration of use and po- tency of dose are factors, or that certain types are more difficult to withdraw from. Some say that genetics, environment, trauma, or psy- chiatric history may play a role. But the truth is, there is little consen- sus, and even less scientific evidence.

> *... age, sex, and the presence or absence of a history of psychiatric, alcoholic, or drug-related problems had no bearing on development of tolerance or withdrawal, thus raising the question about the valid- ity of the "addiction-prone" concept.*[320]

> — Maletzky & Klotter, International Journal of the Addic- tions, 1976

I wish I had a better answer here. Hopefully, future studies will shine a light on it. For right now, the best way to avoid BWS is to not take benzos long-term. Unfortunately, for many of us, it's a little late for that.

Is there anything I can do to help prevent a difficult withdrawal?

Yes. Don't stop cold turkey!

This is a big one. Few rules in benzo withdrawal are as universally accepted as this one. Most experts agree that stopping benzos abruptly is the most dangerous action you can take when on a benzo long-term. A slow taper under a doctor's supervision is the best choice and can significantly reduce complications.

Now, if you CT'd (stopped cold turkey) already, don't fret. Many people have come before you and have managed to have a successful withdrawal and became benzo-free. I'll talk more about this in a little bit.

Stages of Benzo Withdrawal

What are the stages of benzo withdrawal?

Can I just say it one more time? Everybody's different. Whew, that felt good.

Most benzo resources break the withdrawal process into stages, such as acute and protracted withdrawal, and use terms like interdose and tolerance. But some differ. I decided to go with the most common terminology. You may disagree with my stages or their duration, which I understand entirely. Please remember that these are just for organizational purposes used in this book.

Stages of Withdrawal:

- Interdose Withdrawal
- Tolerance Withdrawal
- Taper Withdrawal
- Acute Withdrawal
- Protracted Withdrawal

Time to look at each in detail.

What is Interdose Withdrawal?

Experiencing symptoms between doses of a benzo is called interdose withdrawal. This most commonly occurs in people who are on benzos with a shorter half-life, such as midazolam, oxazepam, and temazepam. It can also occur in people who take benzos periodically, such as before a stressful event like flying or public speaking. Once a person takes his/her next dose, the symptoms usually ease.

What is Tolerance Withdrawal?

After taking benzos for several weeks, your body will start to adapt, and the drug can stop being as effective. Your body has reached stasis and has adjusted to the drug's effects. Therefore, your body craves more of the drug to provide the same benefits, which causes you to increase your dose. If your body doesn't get more of the drug, then it can go into tolerance withdrawal, meaning that your body has reached tolerance of the medication and craves more. Many of the symptoms during this withdrawal phase can be similar to those experienced during and after actual withdrawal of the drug.

What is Taper Withdrawal?

Taper withdrawal is when you experience withdrawal symptoms while reducing your dosage. Tapering slowly can significantly reduce symptoms during this stage. I have identified the time frame for this as six months to two years, although it may take longer for some.

What is Acute Withdrawal?

The acute withdrawal period starts the day after your last dose of benzos, when you're finally benzo-free. Unfortunately, symptoms often continue and even escalate after the taper is completed. Determining the length of the acute phase is where we find some dissension, as I mentioned earlier in this chapter.

According to Ashton, the "pharmacological" benzodiazepine withdrawal syndrome was initially described as lasting anywhere between 5–28 days. Since then, more studies have revealed that withdrawal can last significantly longer. Ashton herself stated, "the duration of this acute phase has probably been underestimated."[321] Most of the initial clinical studies that identified the length of acute withdrawal only lasted for four to eight weeks, so they didn't monitor the patients long enough to know if their symptoms continued.

The website *BenzoBuddies* (www.benzobuddies.com) identifies the transition from acute withdrawal to protracted withdrawal at 18 months, and I think this is a more accurate estimate. Thus, for the purposes of this book, I'll define acute withdrawal as lasting from last dose to 18 months. Remember, this doesn't mean that your acute withdrawal will last 18 months. In fact, the odds are against it. It only means that any withdrawal in that period is still considered acute.

And finally, what is Protracted Withdrawal?

Protracted Withdrawal goes by many names, depending on whom you ask. It's known as protracted withdrawal syndrome (PWS), post-withdrawal, post-withdrawal syndrome (also PWS), prolonged withdrawal syndrome (again, PWS), and persistent withdrawal syndrome (yes, you guessed it, PWS one more time). So, it seems clear that the acronym PWS appears to be universal even if the name changes.

For the purposes of the book, I'll use "protracted withdrawal syndrome" and "PWS" to refer to people who continue to experience withdrawal symptoms past the acute phase. As I just mentioned, I'll identify that cut off time at 18 months. So, if you're still dealing with withdrawal symptoms after the 18-month mark, then you would be in protracted withdrawal. I am quite familiar with this since I am one of these unlucky few.

What causes protracted withdrawal? Why do some get it and others do not?

Prof. Ashton has identified several possible causes of protracted withdrawal. Perhaps the drugs stay in the body longer in some cases and are undetectable in the blood. Or the neurotransmitters develop hyperexcitability, which is very slow to reverse itself after withdrawal. Some, like Prof. Lader, have suggested that there may be neurological damage in the brain that causes the lingering symptoms. Other ideas include damage to the respiratory muscles, learning deficit, memory impairment, PTSD, and even changes to the gut and immune systems. Also, certain types of benzos, such as clonazepam (Klonopin), appear to have a higher incidence of protracted withdrawal than the others in their class.[322]

There are plenty of ideas of what causes protracted withdrawal, but few definite answers.

What are windows and waves?

I like this question. I like it because it's simple. I don't get a whole lot of those.

Basically, a wave is when you experience intense symptoms during withdrawal for a period of time. This can be days, weeks, or even months. Windows are the opposite. A window is when you feel good and most, or all, your symptoms have subsided. You start to feel normal again. Most people with BWS go through windows and waves at some point in their recovery. It may feel much like a roller coaster. Symptoms get better, then they get worse, then they get better, etc. There are even times when some symptoms get worse while other symptoms get better.

What causes the waves?

Waves can be caused by anxiety, stress, diet, alcohol, caffeine, exercise, lack of exercise, etc. Perhaps there was a trigger for the wave, perhaps there wasn't. Many people feel that their waves are just part of the cycle of withdrawal and that there is nothing they can do to prevent them.

My waves still come and go. They're better than they were, but sometimes the strength of a new wave can surprise me. The fun part is that I still don't know what really causes them. I've tried to find a connection to something concrete, but it's fuzzy. Stressful situations, especially ones that last for a week or two, seem to be a factor. Many people say that alcohol, sugar, or caffeine can kick them into waves, but I haven't noticed that connection for me.

The truth is, there is not one answer. We all experience withdrawal differently and will have different causes for the events that happen.

The Taper

So, what about tapering? What is a taper?

According to the Merriam-Webster dictionary, the word taper means "to become progressively smaller toward one end." But perhaps that definition doesn't work for us. Or my favorite one is "to cause to taper." That's not particularly helpful either. The definition that does fit our subject here is "to diminish gradually."[323] As you may have heard by now, it can be dangerous to stop taking benzos abruptly. The better option is to reduce your dosage over a stretched-out period.

I was on 2 mg of clonazepam before I started my taper and I'd been taking the drug for 11 years. I wanted off, and I wanted off immediately. But, thanks to a good doctor and *The Ashton Manual,* I realized that removing benzos from my system was going to take time. Still, going slow wasn't going to be easy. When something inside of you is doing damage to your body, whether perceived or actual, your gut reaction is to remove it as fast as possible. To continually take this drug was a psychological nightmare. I just wanted to stop it now and get over it. It seems contrary to common sense that to be free from benzos, you need to keep taking them. But it's true.

As I discussed earlier, after long-term use of benzos, your body will reach homeostasis. It's used to having benzos in the body and has become reliant on them. Removing them from your system abruptly is a ruthless thing to do to your body. Play nice and allow your body time to catch up.

What if I already CT'd?

If you already stopped taking benzos cold turkey, don't panic. Thousands of people have CT'd and recovered fully — many under doctor's orders. While all evidence points to an easier withdrawal period if you taper slowly, it also points to success even for those who stop more rapidly.

Most of the information in this book applies to those who CT'd just as much as those who taper slowly. Your body is still healing, just like the rest of us, and it will take time. I encourage you to get on the boards and talk with others who have CT'd. You might be surprised at the number of people in the same boat.

So, tell me how I should taper?

See *The Ashton Manual.* And talk to your doc.

That's it. Seriously?

Seriously. I'll touch on a few basics here, but please do not start to taper without reading *The Ashton Manual* and speaking with your doctor. Those two steps are the absolute minimum. But, I am happy to provide some supplemental information, if you wish.

Thanks. So, how long should I taper?

Take as long as you need. There are some general guidelines, but it varies.

> *The precise rate of withdrawal is an individual matter. It depends on many factors including the dose and type of benzodiazepine used, duration of use, personality, lifestyle, previous experience, specific vulnerabilities, and the (perhaps genetically determined) speed of your recovery systems...You may need to resist attempts from outsiders (clinics, doctors) to persuade you into a rapid withdrawal.*[324]
>
> — Prof. Ashton

Think of this as good news. It's up to you. You get to take your time and withdraw at a rate that works for you. Flexibility is the key. It might take several months. It might take a few years. If symptoms are increasing, perhaps you hold steady for a few months at a certain level. Nothing wrong with that.

Some sources say that you shouldn't taper longer than six months. Some even recommend 6–8 weeks. They claim that anything longer just drags out the inevitable and some even claim it increases symptoms. Still, most of the evidence I have seen supports the mantra "slower is better." And, if it takes you a year or two to withdraw, then so be it. I took a year-and-a-half, and I wish in hindsight that I had taken longer.

Still, if you're looking for something more specific, there is a generally accepted guideline for withdrawal that is relatively consistent: "The 10/2 Rule." It's based on the *BenzoBuddies* recommendation of a 10% reduction of the current dose every 1–2 weeks. Keep in mind that the most important thing is to be flexible and go at your own pace.[325]

> *It cannot be too strongly stressed that withdrawal symptoms can be minimised and largely avoided by slow tapering, tailored to the individual's needs.*[326]
>
> — Prof. Ashton

If it gets too hard, can I just increase my dosage for a bit?

Updosing — increasing your dosage temporarily during taper — is not recommended and most agree that it should be avoided, if possible. Evidence shows that people who raised their dosage during taper had a more difficult time withdrawing once they decided to start again. The general rule is to go down in dose or stay put, but don't updose unless your symptoms are unbearable or life-threatening.

Please speak with your doctor if you feel you need to updose to handle your symptoms.

What is kindling?

Kindling is still somewhat of a mystery, but we know it happens. Some people have gone back on benzos for some reason or another once they have become benzo-free. When they decide to withdraw again, it's often harder than it was the first time. This is due to a process known as "kindling." While most of the current resources and support sites clearly say that kindling is an issue, others might not feel it is a significant problem.

> *People who have gone back on benzodiazepines, having failed at the first attempt at withdrawal, can be just as successful at tapering as first-timers.*[327]

— Prof. Ashton

This is another time that I would much rather be safe than sorry. After successfully going through withdrawal, the last thing I would want to do is to go back on the drugs. Even if withdrawing again is no more difficult than it was the first time, do I really want to go through that again? Once I'm benzo-free, I'm staying that way, no matter what.

I have heard terms like "diazepam substitution" and "titration." What do those have to do with tapering?

There is more than one way to taper from benzos. There are options, and you and your doctor will need to decide which one is best for you. Let's look at a few of these here.[328]

Direct Taper - The first and most straightforward method of tapering is a direct taper. This means that you reduce the dosage of the benzodiazepine you're currently on and you don't substitute another benzo, like diazepam. This is the most popular method. You will still need a doctor to prescribe differing doses and perhaps a pill cutter to split pills, but other than that, it's basic. This method works best for benzos that are less potent or have a longer half-life.

Substitution Taper - This method of tapering includes switching, over time, from your benzo to another benzo that is better for tapering. The choice for substitution is usually diazepam (Valium). Diazepam has a long half-life and is less potent, making it a good substitute for a slow tapering schedule. Clonazepam has been used by some physicians, but this is not recommended by many in the benzo community since it binds more tightly to the GABA receptors, is difficult to reduce dosage at lower milligrams, and has a higher incidence of protracted withdrawal complications. Diazepam substitution will take more planning and coordination with your doctor and may extend your tapering time to include switching between benzos, but it has been a very effective method for people who take more potent benzos.

Titration Taper - Titration means mixing benzos with milk or water to create a liquid form of the drug, allowing the user to better control her dosage. This allows for very small and accurate doses. It also allows you to stay on one medication while tapering at a slow, controlled rate.

To learn more about these methods, visit *The Ashton Manual* and the *BenzoBuddies* website.

Did you make mistakes with your taper?

I was on clonazepam for eleven years and then tapered for 18 months before I was benzo-free. In retrospect, that was too fast for me. I should have tapered more slowly.

When I met with Dr. V and discussed my taper schedule, he had a more rapid approach in mind, but I stuck to my guns. I decided to cut .25 mg of clonazepam every two weeks. This is only a 12.5% reduction the first time, which isn't much more than the 10/2 rule of 10%. But that is not where I made the mistake.

The part that I didn't remember was that the reduction needed to be based on the current dose, and not the original dose. Therefore, the first reduction was 0.25 mg from 2 mg, which is 12.5%, but once I got down to 1 mg, I was cutting my dosage at a rate of 25%. And when I got to 0.5 mg, I was reducing my dose at a rate of 50%. No surprise that I had more problems as I moved further down on my taper schedule.

One of the challenges I faced was the limited dosage amounts available for clonazepam. The smallest pill I could get was 0.5 mg. I had a pill cutter that allowed me to cut it in half, but anything smaller than that was difficult. Therefore, 0.25 mg was my smallest reasonable reduction without switching to diazepam or using titration.

I did my best with what I knew at the time, but I do hope that others can learn from my mistakes.

CHAPTER 12

THE SYMPTOMS

Is this where we get to talk about all the withdrawal symptoms?

This is the place. Any questions before I dive in?

If you had to use just one word to convey the general experience of this cluster of symptoms, what would it be?

Hypersensitivity.

Those of us in benzo withdrawal feel more — more pain, more agitation, more restlessness, more emotion, more aches, more spasms, more anxiety, more depression, more hopelessness.

Benzo dependence has caused our central nervous systems to become hypersensitive and over-reactive to everyday stimuli. Imagine drinking one cup of coffee but reacting like you drank five. Or even ten. A work party might induce mild anxiety in the average person. Imagine if that same event felt like you were speaking in front of a thousand people. Naked. Imagine being dog tired but inside your body energy is shooting through and your muscles are spasming as if you just drank a six-pack of Red Bull.

Sounds fun, right? And sensitivity is just the tip of the iceberg. Add depersonalization, memory and cognitive dysfunction, muscle tightness and spasms, heart palpitations, phantom nerve sensations, and chronic gastrointestinal distress.

Now, before you freak out, please remember that while those examples are real, they're also extremes. I'm using them here to make a point.

What if my symptoms are permanent?

As I discussed earlier, it's possible. I wish I could say otherwise. But it's also unlikely. Thousands of people have gone down this path before you. The majority say that they fully healed, eventually. The biggest complaint was how long it took.

I still have symptoms, but I am doing so much better than I was. In fact, much of that improvement has happened in just the past six months. Now, wouldn't it make sense that this trend will continue? Especially, when most people say it will.

> All the evidence shows that a steady decline in symptoms almost invariably continues after withdrawal, though it can take a long time — even several years in some cases.[329]

— Prof. Ashton

When you freak out that your belly, memory, skin condition, or muscles will never return to normal, take a pause and tell yourself that the odds are significantly in your favor that you will heal. I can't promise you that you won't have permanent damage, but I also can't guarantee that you won't get hit by a bus tomorrow. As you start to heal, focus on how far you have come from your worst days. Remember that and know that the trend will continue, even if it takes a while.

So, where do we start?

Prof. Ashton divides symptoms into two high-level categories: psychological and physical. Let's stick with her classification for our discussion.

Psychological Symptoms include:[330]

- **Anxiety** - General (GAD), Hypochondria, Panic Attacks, Paranoid Thoughts, Phobias
- **Behavioral** - Anger, Irritability, Aggression, Depression,

Obsessions, Suicidal Thoughts
- **Cognitive** - Cognitive Dysfunction, Memory Dysfunction, Intrusive Memories
- **Excitability** - Akathisia, Jumpiness, Restlessness, Restless Legs
- **Perception** - Depersonalization, Derealization, Hallucinations, Misperceptions, Perceptual Distortions
- **Sleeping** - Insomnia, Nightmares
- **Social** - Agoraphobia, Social Phobias

Anxiety Symptoms

I guess we should start with anxiety then.

Great choice. If you had to pick a single "core" symptom associated with benzo withdrawal, it would have to be anxiety and its related variations. This shouldn't be a surprise to anyone since benzos are classified as anti-anxiety drugs.

What are the primary anxiety symptoms in withdrawal?

Generalized Anxiety - People with Generalized Anxiety Disorder (GAD) often experience chronic, consistent worry about a variety of issues and concerns. This is the most common form of anxiety. According to the Anxiety and Depression Association of America (ADAA), GAD affects about 6.8 million adults in the U.S., but only 43% are receiving treatment.[331]

Hypochondria - Hypochondria is also known as hypochondriasis, illness anxiety disorder, or somatic symptoms disorder and it's often identified by constant worrying about one's own health. This is perhaps the most frightening type of anxiety during withdrawal due to the continuous barrage of physical aches, pains, sensations, and perceptions that give an obsessive mind plenty of ammunition.

Panic Attacks - Panic disorder (PD) affects 2-3% of the U.S. population, and the attacks often occur without warning.[332] Prof. Ashton states, "Panic attacks may appear for the first time during withdrawal, although some patients have long experience with this distressing symptom." Ashton also reminds patients that these rarely last longer than half-an-hour and are never fatal.[333]

Paranoid Thoughts - Normal anxious thoughts are often confused as paranoia. Clinical paranoia is identified as experiencing consistent, ongoing suspicions that are unfair and unrealistic. Paranoid thoughts, like jealousy, conspiracy theories, and the feeling that others are out to get you, can be elevated during withdrawal.

Phobias - The list of identified and named phobias numbers in the hundreds. Many are familiar with the more common ones, such as acrophobia, agoraphobia, claustrophobia, and one of the most popular in Hollywood, arachnophobia. In benzo withdrawal, preexisting phobias can escalate, and new phobias can emerge.

Is the anxiety in withdrawal similar to what many of us had prior to benzos?

It's similar but often stronger.

It makes sense that any of us who had anxiety issues before benzos should expect that anxiety to return once we start to remove the drug from our bodies. And it does. But it often reappears in a highly elevated state. Some people complain that anxiety was two, three, four, even five times worse than they experienced before.

Damage to the GABA receptors is a likely culprit here, which makes it more difficult for us to calm ourselves down from an anxiety-driven state. But, it's not just the return of anxiety that is the trigger here. Even patients who took benzos for insomnia or other conditions and never had a struggle with anxiety can develop mild to moderate anxiety issues upon withdrawal.

What are the most common anxiety symptoms in withdrawal?

Hypochondria. I shared my experiences with it earlier, but I'm not the only one. Even someone without heightened anxiety would obsess about all these crazy things happening to his/her body. And unfortunately, hypochondria and its more contemporary sibling "cyberchondria," take a significant financial toll. In Britain, 20% of all National Health Service (NHS) appointments are taken up by hypochondriacs.

Some say that Internet searching, in addition to the use of fitness trackers, is partly responsible for the recent increase. Anxiety about our health is reported to cost the NHS upwards of £420 million a year.[334]

What was your experience with anxiety in withdrawal?

Anxiety was one of my strongest withdrawal symptoms and by far the scariest. I experienced generalized anxiety, hypochondria, phobias, and occasional panic attacks. Although I had mild issues with anxiety in the past, this was so much worse. There were times I was petrified of everything. Even the smallest, most trivial things could send my mind ruminating on worse-case scenario outcomes. It's crazy, and I hated being that way. But I was that way, and I had to learn to deal with it.

Hypochondria was my worst, as I already mentioned. I had chronic fears that something more serious was wrong, but time after time I would have to step back, calm myself down, and realize that it's just benzo withdrawal. Panic attacks were another big surprise for me. I don't believe that I ever had a panic attack before benzo withdrawal. It's a terrifying ordeal, and I would be happy if I never have another one again. Phobias were also part of my anxiety symptom collection.

How did you handle your anxiety symptoms?

I did what so many of us do, I used avoidance. I avoided anything I could that might trigger an anxious episode. Since our reactions are so severe to certain triggers during this time, and since so often one obsession can escalate and lead to others, I found it helpful to avoid stimuli that I couldn't handle in my current state. And this included isolation. Since I was unable to work in an office for a while, I became isolated. I worked on the book and spent time in my home with my wife. She also works from home, so we created our own little world. It's quiet, safe, and cozy and it has allowed me time to heal. But avoidance and isolation are not true long-term solutions.

I didn't know it at the beginning, but I had built a protective bubble. Sometimes I refer to it as my box, cocoon, or even prison cell.

However you look at it, it's very restrictive. And my bubble got smaller and smaller the more anxiety I felt. I limited my exposure to friends and even family. I didn't fly at all. I didn't travel without making sure I could control every aspect of the trip. I disconnected from almost all news, especially stories about health, politics, and anything else that irritated me — which was just about everything.

While that helped for a while, the bubble never stopped shrinking. It was never enough. I could lock the door and avoid the world for just so long. It helps for a while, but at some point, I had to face the world again. I finally made the decision that I needed to grow my bubble instead of shrinking it. So, I did, and I'm still doing that today. It's a struggle at times, but I just keep reminding myself that I'm retraining my brain to live in the real world. It's my own little version of exposure therapy.

Anxiety is real. Anyone who has suffered it can tell you that. And anxiety during benzo withdrawal, well, it's like anxiety on caffeine, speed, and cocaine all at the same time. If this sounds like you, protect yourself when you need, but know when enough is enough. Take responsibility for your healing and slowly start to get back out there to face the world. It's an amazing, colorful, beautiful, scary, and exciting world and it's just waiting for us.

Behavioral Symptoms

What are the primary behavioral symptoms of withdrawal?

Anger/Irritability/Aggression - During benzo withdrawal, our calming mechanism has been damaged, which can make it more difficult for us to control our feelings of anger, aggression, and rage. This experience is sometimes referred to as "benzo rage." This lack of control can lead to physical violence and abuse. It's vital when dealing with this type of issue that we protect those at risk of harm. But it's also important to maintain compassion and understanding for those who may not be able to regulate their responses due to the effects of withdrawal. These situations are delicate and need to be handled with compassion and understanding for all those involved.

Depression/Suicidal Thoughts - Depression is quite common during benzo withdrawal. While it may not be a direct effect of the benzos, the suffering many endure could in of itself cause the onset of moderate to severe depressive episodes. Depression can lead to suicidal thoughts during withdrawal, and these thoughts need to be taken seriously and managed with therapy, medication, and support, as needed. Many, including myself, started taking an anti-depressant before or during withdrawal to help manage depressive symptoms. Even though drugs like SSRIs are another medication that may need to be withdrawn from later, sometimes this course of action is the best solution during this challenging time. Please consult with your doctor or therapist if you feel you need help.

Obsessions - Obsessive traits, such as OCD, may be increased during withdrawal. It's important to remember the cause of this increase and know that they will usually decrease as we start to heal.

How did you handle your anger and irritability during withdrawal?

Most psychiatric professionals will agree that the only difference between the average person on the street and a homicidal killer is the ability to regulate our impulses of anger, aggression, and even hatred. These are normal emotions in every human being. Men, women, children — we all feel hostility and even rage at times in our lives. Yes, I experienced these emotions during withdrawal. In fact, I'm dealing with them right now as I write this. I have been struggling with ongoing anger and depression based on a variety of triggers in my life.

I realized early on that my problems with anger weren't caused by just one issue. I've been getting mad at all sorts of things going on around me, whether in the news, online, or even within my own neighborhood. My problem isn't the trigger; it's my reaction. So, I've established some boundaries. Since my emotions are so raw during withdrawal, I need to make sure that I don't get irritated so easily. It's a temporary fix, but I need to manage the best I can with what abilities I have at the time.

During my research, I came across a book titled *The Subtle Art of*

Not Giving a F*ck by Mark Manson. Great title, I know. Anyway, this book surprised me and really challenged my thinking in a few areas. In his book, Manson challenges our personal value systems. I never really thought about my values or questioned that they may be wrong. But he asks us to take a hard look at our personal values, evaluate where they came from, and see if it's time for a change.

> *And because you and I and everybody else all have differing needs and personal histories and life circumstances, we will all inevitably come to differing "correct" answers about what our lives mean and how they should be lived.*[335]

— Mark Manson

So, I looked inside myself. I questioned my values. If my value system can't stand up to a bit of self-reflection, then how solid is it, really? At the end of the day, I realized that the other person who makes me so irate just has different values than I do. They're not wrong, and I'm not right — we're just different. We both are struggling to make sense of this crazy world that we live in. We're all just doing our best.

This didn't magically make my anger disappear, but it did help if even just a little. It's only one of several books I've read lately about anger, and each one has taught me a new lesson that I have added to my toolbox. It's something, and I'll take every positive change I can get.

What about depression?

It just makes sense. Anyone who goes through hardships like benzo withdrawal will probably struggle with some form of depression. I took an anti-depressant a couple of times prior to starting my withdrawal, more as a preventive measure than anything else. I stopped taking the fluoxetine (Prozac) due to an adverse reaction, and I ended the citalopram (Celexa) because I didn't want another medication inside of me messing things up.

Eventually, I managed my moods with meditation, counseling, exercise, and reading. There were days, weeks, even months when I was moderately to severely depressed, but with my tools and support system, I got through it.

Cognitive Symptoms

What are the primary cognitive symptoms of withdrawal?

Cognitive/Memory Dysfunction - Poor memory and cognitive dysfunction are two common and very distressing side effects of benzo withdrawal. A couple of studies in 1994 provided some interesting information. The first study, published in *International Clinical Psychopharmacology*, found that many benzo patients were cognitively impaired ten months after withdrawal as compared to control groups. In fact, many users complained that it took years before their previous mental capacity returned.[336]

The second study, published in *Psychological Medicine*, detailed similar effects:

> *The main cognitive functions assessed in this study include working memory, verbal learning and memory, visuo-motor and visuo-conceptual skills. The lack of evidence for clinically significant cognitive recovery raises concern about the severity and reversibility of any underlying BZ-induced organic impairment.*[337]

Some Swedish studies have discovered that intellectual impairment, although improved, was still present four to six years after cessation.[338]

Intrusive Memories - Another very uncomfortable cognitive side effect can be intrusive memories. These can be traumatic events from someone's past or even a vivid memory of another person they haven't seen or thought about for years. One theory is that this is linked to dreaming. Since benzos affect REM sleep and often prevent dreaming during their use, this could be a sign of healing, and that normal dreaming is starting to return.

I'm concerned about memory loss. Did you experience this?

As I write this section, I am unemployed. I ended my last two database contracts because of my inability to perform well enough mentally in the high-stress technical field of information technology (IT). As I mentioned earlier, my difficulties with memory and cognitive functioning make it hard to keep up, especially when new technical skills are involved.

So, I'm at home most days now writing this book. It's a labor of love, but a difficult struggle at times. My memory comes and goes and creates hurdles. I can't count the number of times I have read, notated, and registered one article and then found that I already logged it a few days prior with absolutely no recollection of it. Still, writing is better suited to my current cognitive state than IT, and I'm happy to have it to keep me busy.

The mental struggles still irritate me now and then, but I do believe it's slowly getting better. Perhaps I can return to database work soon so I can help pay the bills for the house. That is until this book is published and becomes an international bestseller. Big dreams, huh?

Is there anything I can do to help prevent this, or manage it better?

I believe the best thing you can do to maintain your cognitive function is to keep using your brain. Stay as mentally active as you can during withdrawal. It's the old "use it or lose it" rule. Learn a new skill or hobby. Take a class. Read. Study a new language. Do crossword puzzles, or word searches, or Sudoku, or whatever rocks your boat. Researching this book was a saving grace for me during withdrawal. It kept me busy and gave me a purpose.

Physical activity is also important. Exercise provides oxygen-rich blood to your brain, which keeps it energized, growing, and healing. I don't mean you have to push yourself hard, especially when you're having a bad day. But do what you can. Even a 10-minute walk helps.

Keeping socially active with your family and friends can also help. It's your brain, and it's trying to repair itself — give it all the help you can.

Excitability Symptoms

What do you mean by excitability symptoms?

Let's backtrack just for a second. Benzos are classified as minor tranquilizers, and so they effectively calm the body down when used. When we remove them from our systems, this calming effect goes away. Also, the GABA receptors are left in a diminished capacity for receiving any calming messages. Therefore, our bodies respond on the inside as if we've been attacked even though we may appear calm and relaxed on the outside.

The common forms of excitability in withdrawal include akathisia, jumpiness, and restlessness.

What is akathisia?

Simply put, akathisia is a disorder where the patient has a feeling of inner restlessness and the urgency to keep moving. It's like being on high doses of caffeine all the time, even when you're trying to sleep. You just want to get up and do something, like run a marathon or even climb the stairs. Anything to keep moving. Akathisia is a common side effect of earlier anti-psychotic drugs, and you guessed it, of benzos too.

Did you experience this?

This is a big one for me. It's better now, but I still struggle with it. I get it mostly when I try to nap or in the evening when I'm trying to relax or watch TV. Sometimes it's just a sense of urgency to move, sometimes it's an internal vibration, and sometimes, when I'm trying to sleep, it feels like a tiny jackhammer inside of my bones.

I can't count the number of times that I have had to get up and go do something even though I desperately wanted to just sit and rest. My go-to solution is practicing the drums. I have a couple of drum kits in the basement that I'd play for an hour or so, and then I usually feel better. Sometimes I just walk up and down the steps. If it's nice outside and not too late, I'll go for a walk.

The fact that the akathisia increases when I'm tired is the most frustrating part. Getting a good night's sleep is a struggle. How do you nap or sleep at night if your body is still running a marathon inside? I would frequently fall asleep and then jolt myself awake. Then I'd fall asleep again. Lather. Rinse. Repeat.

On the bright side, it's a symptom that my wife can see. Unlike rashes or benzo belly, most of the symptoms of BWS are invisible to others. And since many people still think we're making this up, it's nice to have a visible symptom. So, when my wife tells me in the morning that I was jittery and jolting throughout the night, at least I have a witness. It's not a big win, but I'll take it.

Restlessness and restless legs are all a part of the same issue. In fact, it's my legs that are the most agitated when I'm trying to relax in the evening. Jumpiness or reactive movements are also linked and common in withdrawal.

Perception Symptoms

Could you explain perception symptoms?

Let me break out the primary perception symptoms to help explain it here:

Depersonalization/Derealization - Both disorders are related to feeling detached from reality. Depersonalization is feeling detached from yourself as if you're viewing yourself from outside your body. Derealization is feeling disconnected from your surroundings, almost like you're living in a dreamlike state. Vertigo and lightheadedness are also common with derealization.

According to Prof. Ashton, derealization and depersonalization are most frequent with rapid withdrawal from benzos, and especially with withdrawal from clonazepam (Klonopin).[339] Some experts believe that it's a defense mechanism that helps the body cope with excessive suffering by detaching from the experience.

Hallucinations - Hallucinations are perhaps the most terrifying of all possible symptoms. They're more common in people attempting rapid detox from benzos and are very uncommon with a slow taper. Treatment usually involves helping the patient recognize that the hallucination is unreal, which aids in alleviating the fear.

Misperceptions and perceptual distortions can also be symptoms of benzo withdrawal.

Don't tell me you have experience with these too.

Thankfully, I don't. I dealt with vertigo, which sometimes is associated with derealization. Since I will cover that later, I won't go into detail here. I sympathize with those who deal with these symptoms, and I am grateful that this is an area where I have no direct experience.

Still, several people have shared their stories with me. Derealization is often connected to depersonalization but can occur separately. With depersonalization, many people say they can look in the mirror but don't recognize themselves. The world around them feels threatening and unsafe. Some say it's as if being trapped in a fog.

Cognitive behavioral therapy and psychodynamic therapy are conventional treatments for these conditions. They help the patient understand the causes and learn techniques to help deal with the symptoms, so the patient can feel more connected to their feelings and the world around them.[340] Therapy, in addition to medication, is the standard treatment for hallucinations.

Sleeping Symptoms

How common is insomnia in benzo withdrawal?

Insomnia is one of the most common complaints during benzo withdrawal.

Sleep helps us heal, but we often can't sleep well during withdrawal. This makes our symptoms worse, which then makes it harder to sleep — see a pattern? It's estimated that between 30 and 40 million Americans have trouble sleeping each night.[341] So, if you have trouble sleeping, you're in good company.

Since benzos are frequently used as a treatment for insomnia, it makes sense that withdrawal from the drug could affect a person's ability to sleep. The sleep that people experience while taking benzos is not a typical, healthy type of sleep. Benzos inhibit both REM (rapid eye movement) sleep and SWS (slow wave sleep), so you don't get the deep sleep that your body really needs.

Another common sleep symptom of withdrawal is nightmares. During withdrawal, many patients experience very vivid dreams and nightmares. As I mentioned earlier, this may be a sign of recovery. The dream process was subdued during benzo use and now is starting to return to its normal functioning. The nightmares usually subside in a couple of months once the body adjusts to normal REM sleep.[342]

What was your experience with this?

Insomnia is one of my lingering symptoms. Only about a month ago, I started to average six hours of sleep a night, and I must tell you, it's the most fantastic thing. I hope it lasts, but at least it's a sign that I can get back to a regular sleep pattern. At some stages of withdrawal, I averaged three to four hours a night and had many sleepless nights. Still do now and then. I know some people who say they have been wide awake for almost a week.

One of the more unsettling — and yet welcome — changes for me was the return of dreams. For years, my wife would share her dreams with me in the morning. I always felt left out of this conversation. I rarely remembered my dreams, to the point of wondering if I dreamed at all. After withdrawal, though, things changed. I now realize that the clonazepam suppressed my dreaming for over 12 years. Now I dream. I even remember my dreams from time to time and get a chance to share them with my wife. I no longer feel left out.

Any suggestions to help with sleep?

Unfortunately, the most popular (short-term) medications for insomnia are z-drugs and other benzodiazepines, and I can't say I'd recommend those for obvious reasons. Other medications might help, but they can have their own side effects and issues. Some people have had success with the hormone melatonin, but it also has potential side effects, including possible withdrawal complications. I tried Advil PM for a few months in the middle of acute withdrawal, which carries the same antihistamine (diphenhydramine) as Benadryl. It worked for me in the short-term, but eventually, I had to discontinue it because it made my akathisia even worse and I was concerned about long-term side effects.

Eventually, I focused on more natural methods to help me sleep. Here are some suggestions I found useful:

- **Avoid eating before bed** - Large meals at or near bedtime can keep you awake.
- **Be active** - Having a mentally and physically active day tires out your body and mind.
- **Cognitive Behavioral Therapy (CBT)** - CBT has been found successful for many with insomnia by helping the patient control or eliminate negative thoughts. CBT is found in most studies to be as effective — if not more so — than most medications.
- **Cool off** - Cooling off your body temperature triggers a good night sleep. Open a window if you can.
- **Don't worry** - Try not to worry about sleep. Remember, you are healing. Getting anxious about not sleeping only makes the problem worse. Be kind to yourself and know that your body will eventually adjust.
- **Get up** - Lying in bed and ruminating is not very productive. That's when my brain drifts to dark places. Get up and do something for one hour, then return and try again. Sometimes that will reset your internal clock and clear your mind.
- **Keep to a routine** - We all have a sleep cycle, and when it gets disrupted it can cause problems.
- **Limit caffeine, alcohol, and nicotine** - Most medical professionals recommend that you avoid these drugs, especially close to bedtime.
- **Remove screens from the bedroom** - Screen time (TV, phone, tablet) before bed hinders your ability to sleep. The blue light emitted from these electronic devices can disrupt the body's circadian rhythm and suppress the body's natural release of melatonin, which is essential for helping you sleep. I try to avoid screen time within two hours of bed.

By developing some of these good sleep habits, you might find you get some of the shut-eye you so desperately need.

Social Symptoms

What are the social symptoms of withdrawal?

The Diagnostic and Statistical Manual of Mental Disorders (DSM) divides social anxiety into two specific sub-types: Those with specific social anxiety have anxiety in very specific settings, environments, or conditions, such as public speaking. People with general social anxiety have trouble in almost any social situation.[343]

Social anxiety is a widespread problem for people on benzos. Many started taking the drug because of this issue, and others developed it during the process. It can be very frightening and extremely limiting. I've chatted online with far too many people who can barely leave their houses, let alone meet with people in a public setting. Social anxiety issues rob people of their freedom.

Okay, I must ask, knowing the answer. But did you have experience with social symptoms?

Actually, no. Well, not really.

For me, social anxiety has never been an issue. I can, and have, spoken in front of a thousand plus people without breaking a sweat. I have plenty of fears, as you might have figured out by now, but I am quite thankful that social anxiety is not one of them.

Still, during withdrawal, I did get a tiny taste of what others may have felt. Just a taste. Compared to those who really suffer from this condition, my experience was mild at best. I have felt some anxiety and restlessness when others are around, and I occasionally freeze up in some conversations. It's a problem that I never had before. Part of my issue might be that I am out of practice due to my self-inflicted isolation. Clearly, my social skills have atrophied. I don't really know the cause, but it has given me a small taste of social anxiety, and I'm very grateful that it's not a fear that I must live with every day.

Any suggestions to those who do suffer?

One of the most successful treatments for social anxiety has been cognitive-behavioral therapy (CBT), just as it is for insomnia. This requires time and the support of a good psychologist or psychiatrist, but it's perhaps the most effective long-term solution for managing the condition.

Medications, such as antidepressants, can have some effect in the management of social anxiety but have not shown to have the same success as therapy over time. Group support has been shown to be helpful, especially in conjunction with therapy. I'd encourage you to speak with your doctor or therapist if you wish to pursue these avenues of treatment.

There are other self-help treatments for social anxiety, such as self-help books, relaxation, deep breathing exercises, and self-lead exposure therapy. It's completely understandable that you might tend to close-off from the outside world to protect yourself during benzo withdrawal, but just remember that at some point you may want to rejoin the social world. The further isolated you become, the harder that task may be.

What about the physical symptoms?

Physical symptoms include:[344]

- **Abdominal/Gastrointestinal** - Abdominal Pain, Appetite Change, Benzo Belly, Constipation, Diarrhea, Distention, Inflammation, Nausea, Groin Pain, Menstrual Difficulties, Pelvic Floor Dysfunction, Urinary Difficulties, Vomiting, Weight Change
- **Eyes, Ears, Nose & Mouth** - Blurred Vision, Double Vision, Difficulty Swallowing, Dry Mouth, Metallic Taste, Oral Thrush, Sore Eyes, Dry Eyes, Sound & Light Sensitivity, Tinnitus, Unusual Smell
- **Head & Neck** - Balance Issues, Dizziness, Light Headedness, Headache, Neck Pain, Slurred Speech, Throat Tightening
- **Heart & Lungs** - Flushing, Sweating, Heart Palpitations, Over-breathing
- **Muscular** - Aches and Pain, Electric Shocks, Fatigue, Sprains, Pulls, Tears, Stiffness, Tremors, Twitches, Jerks, Tics, Weakness, Convulsions, Paralysis, Seizures

- **Nerve Sensations** - Altered Sensations, Hypersensitivity, Numbness, Paresthesia, Skin Rashes, Itching, Tingling
- **Immune & Endocrine** - Increased Infections, Breast Swelling, Menstrual Difficulties

I'll elaborate on all these next.

Abdominal / Gastrointestinal Symptoms

Okay, what are the primary abdominal symptoms experienced during withdrawal?

Most of us know that our gut takes a big hit during withdrawal. This makes sense because our central nervous system (CNS) is closely linked with our digestive system. So, the list of symptoms below shouldn't be too much of surprise.

Abdominal Pain - Pain in the abdominal area is quite common during withdrawal. The cause is not always known, but most of the time it appears to be related to the gastrointestinal tract. It can range from a mild nuisance to severe pain and seems to be influenced by diet, anxiety, and the randomness of withdrawal waves.

Appetite/Weight Change - Ashton has stated that considerable weight loss (8–10 lbs. or more) can occur during withdrawal.[345] Since benzos can increase appetite, this might be a rebound effect. Gastric distress might also be a cause since many people are forced to adapt their diet to manage symptoms.

Constipation - Constipation can occur during withdrawal and is often aggravated by over-breathing, which I explain in more detail in an upcoming section. Natural laxatives can help with this condition.

Distension/Inflammation - One of the most surprising and frightening symptoms of withdrawal can be abdominal distension. Both men and women have experienced significant and sometimes painful distension, to the point of appearing to be in a late stage of pregnancy. This is usually experienced in conjunction with digestive difficulties, which causes inflammation. It's not a permanent condition, and changes in diet can help manage it.

Gastritis/Diarrhea/Nausea/Vomiting - Due to the effect that withdrawal has on the overall digestive system, other symptoms, such as diarrhea, nausea, and vomiting may not be a surprise. Symptoms common with irritable bowel syndrome, gastritis, acid reflux, and other digestive difficulties are also quite prevalent.

Groin Pain - The upper abdomen is not the only location to experience pain during withdrawal. The groin area can be affected too. Inflammation of the gut can affect the lower abdomen and groin. Factors that also come into play include chronic muscle tightness and injury.

Menstrual Difficulties - Benzos and benzodiazepine withdrawal can play havoc with a woman's menstrual cycle, including heavier bleeding, irregular periods, cessation of periods, bleeding between cycles, and increased breast pain. Women do need to be cautious of anemia and other complications during this time if their cycles become too frequent. There are some connections between progesterone and the GABA receptors that may attribute to this.

Pelvic Floor Dysfunction - Pelvic floor dysfunction has been a common diagnosis in women for some time and is rapidly becoming more common in men as well. It can be aggravated by, or even first appear, during withdrawal. Due to effects that benzo withdrawal has on the tightness of our muscles and on inflammation in the abdomen, this is not unforeseen.

Urinary Difficulties - Increased urinary frequency can be common with benzo withdrawal. Urgency, leaking, and even inability to urinate are also prevalent.

I've heard of something called "benzo belly." Is that related to what you're describing here?

Digestive distress during withdrawal is so prevalent that it even has its own name: "benzo belly." Clever, isn't it? Benzo belly refers to the whole compilation of symptoms of the digestive tract that are the result of benzo use and withdrawal. Some people have no problems at all with digestion during withdrawal, while others have chronic discomfort and wind up on a very limited diet. Many of the symptoms are similar to those associated with irritable bowel syndrome, including nausea, vomiting, diarrhea, constipation, abdominal pain, flatulence, and heartburn.

One of the most visible signs of benzo belly is the belly itself. Distention and inflammation of the gut are common in patients suffering from benzo belly and can be quite noticeable, as I mentioned earlier.

What about food intolerances?

Some people have been known to develop or increase their intolerances to certain foods during withdrawal, even though allergy tests rarely show positive results. Possible factors may include the large number of GABA receptors in the digestive tract, an increase in anxiety-related distress, and even hyperventilation. Diet and anxiety management appear to be the most effective measures of calming benzo belly. Many people have reduced their diets down to just two or three foods for a while so they could avoid the distress.

Did you have issues with benzo belly or any of the other related symptoms?

As I mentioned briefly before, I have had chronic digestive problems for most of my life. Thankfully, I went through my complete taper without any new digestive problems, and I was happy to say that I did not have to add that symptom to my ever-growing list. Unfortunately, I spoke too soon.

After being benzo-free for a few months, I started to have new stomach issues. My diet became more and more restricted. I had already cut out alcohol and caffeine, and then I added sugar to my limitations. I lived off chicken with white rice for a while since it was the only thing that would settle. There were days when my stomach would churn all day long, and nothing would calm it down. Abdominal pain was quite common and severely limited my physical activity. I couldn't get too far from the bathroom, and I found myself more and more house-bound every day. Once the abdomen is inflamed and irritated, a variety of symptoms can be aggravated, including localized pain, distension, inflammation, muscle tightness, urinary difficulties, and general pelvic floor dysfunction.

While I could attribute my stomach churning, cramping, and pain to benzo belly, the chronic pain in my groin and lower abdomen was more of a mystery to me. After all kinds of tests and examinations, including some strong drugs and incorrect diagnosis of prostatitis among others, I developed a theory as to the contributing factors for my lower abdominal distress. Considering my vast amount of education in the field of medicine (basically none), my theory is just that — a theory.

I believe I was suffering from pelvic floor dysfunction aggravated by hyperactive nerves, constant abdominal inflammation, chronic muscle tightness, and gastric distress; all of which have been caused or irritated by benzodiazepine withdrawal. After a series of doctors, physical therapists, and my ongoing experience with these symptoms for over three years, it's the only diagnosis that makes sense to me. But still, it's just a guess.

I did learn another valuable lesson from this experience. When I first started to have groin and abdominal pain my doctor diagnosed me with prostatitis and prescribed Ciprofloxacin HCL. I took the drug without thinking twice about it. Another mistake on my part. I figured it was an antibiotic and I've had antibiotics before so why would there be a problem?

Unfortunately, Ciprofloxacin is part of the class of antibiotics called fluoroquinolones, or quinolones. It wasn't until I was writing this book that I saw a warning about these drugs in *The Ashton Manual*. The quinolones can have an antagonistic effect on the same GABA receptors that have been damaged by the benzos.[346] I believe that this is just another factor that may have aggravated my withdrawal and caused my protracted symptoms.

Anyway, most of my digestive symptoms have eased and are getting better every day.

Did you find anything that helped you with the benzo belly issues?

The most consistent solution that I've learned from people struggling with benzo belly, and one that helped me, was a limited diet. By limiting your diet and removing food types that appear to cause issues, most people find they can control their symptoms enough to get through this stage until their gut fully heals. But I would approach this with caution since a limited diet can cause a nutrition deficiency.

Just like most things with withdrawal, you need to find out what works for you. It really is different for each person. And the only way to find out is through trial and error. The most common food types that people reduce are sugar, caffeine, and alcohol. Start with those and work your way down.

I also found success with kefir milk. I'd never heard of it before withdrawal, but someone suggested it to me on the benzo boards, and I was desperate, so I gave it a chance. For those who are not familiar, kefir grains are a yeast/bacterial fermentation starter and can be used to make probiotic water, milk, and other substances.

So, I tried kefir milk. And I must say it worked. I now drink eight ounces of kefir milk every morning, and my stomach has settled significantly. I even stopped taking Prilosec, a stomach medication which I had been on for over a decade. I still experience problems now and then, but the constant churning has eased, and I'm back on a far more normal diet. I still limit sugar, caffeine, and alcohol, but those are just good overall health habits that I learned and decided to continue.

I'm just using kefir milk as an example here, and I'm not suggesting that it will work for anyone else. Some people have even said that it made their symptoms worse. All fermented beverages may contain small amounts of alcohol, and this includes kefir. If this is a concern of yours, please do your own research before experimenting. Perhaps something else will be the magical elixir to help you through these trying times. Talk to your doctor and/or nutritionist to see what works for you.

Symptoms of the Eyes, Ears, Nose & Mouth

That's an odd collection. Tell me about them.

There is a whole cadre of symptoms that can affect these areas. Here are a few:

Blurred/Double Vision - Some people suffer from vision problems during withdrawal. Benzo withdrawal can affect the eye muscles, which can lead to distorted vision or even eyelid spasms.

Difficulty Swallowing - This can be quite distressing and may even feel like a choking sensation at times. The best course of action is to eat slowly, take small bites, and chew your food thoroughly.

Dry Mouth/Metallic Taste - People can experience dry mouth during benzo withdrawal. It's usually a mild issue but can lead to other problems of the mouth. A metallic taste is also typical.

Oral Thrush - Oral thrush (Oropharyngeal Candidiasis) happens when candida yeast spreads into the mouth. It can appear as white spots inside the mouth, but often the area infected just becomes red and sore. It is common in people with weakened immune systems, the elderly, and newborns. Candida is naturally occurring in different parts of the human body, including your gut. Thrush can happen when the bacteria increases in your digestive system and causes a condition known as candida overgrowth. Avoiding foods with gluten, sugar, and some dairy products can help. If this issue is severe, your doctor can prescribe an antifungal medication.

Sore/Dry Eyes - Some people complain of dry eyes during withdrawal, often in conjunction with dry sinus and mucous membranes.

Sound & Light Sensitivity - It's not uncommon for people in benzo withdrawal to say they have an extreme sensitivity to sounds and light. Our nervous systems have become hyper-excited and can over-react to regular everyday stimulation. Some people have been forced to isolate themselves in their homes to avoid this sensation.

Tinnitus - Tinnitus is very common in benzo withdrawal. Constant or periodic ringing or noise in the ears can range from a mild annoyance to very distressing. There are other possible causes of tinnitus, so if it's severe, it may be wise to visit a specialist to get checked out.

Unusual Smell - The olfactory senses can also be affected by withdrawal. Some people speak of a burned smell. Most of the time there are no external causes for these sensations. Some people even have smells return with the reconnection to lost memories.

I must ask; did you have experience with these symptoms?

Of the symptoms listed above, I can honestly state that I have experienced difficulty swallowing, oral thrush, tinnitus, eyelid spasms, and unusual smell. The good news for me is that two of them, difficulty swallowing and unusual smell, have abated. I have not had any experience with them in months. Some of the others have lingered but are mostly mild now.

Of all the ones listed above, the one that is most common — and most irritating — is the tinnitus. I have two types: One is a distant background hiss that is chronic, but just a mild nuisance most of the time. The second one is an occasional high-pitched, piercing sound. It can be a constant sound or a pulsing one in rhythm with my heartbeat. Sometimes I can ignore it, and sometimes I can't. Since I have been dealing with this issue for a couple of years, I've become somewhat accustomed to it. Then again, there are days...

What about swallowing?

This one was infrequent but quite distressing. I would get some food caught in the back of my throat, and I just couldn't swallow it. Bizarre, and at times frightening. Not to be gross, but I would have to relax and try to cough it back into my mouth and chew it further. Sometimes it would feel like I was going to choke, but thankfully I never did.

And smell?

This is a weird one. I would often get the smell of sage or something similar in my nose. It happened over a six-month period during withdrawal and has not returned. I asked my wife if she could smell it too, but she never did. While it was a relatively benign symptom, I am still glad that it's gone.

Symptoms of the Head & Neck

What are the symptoms of the head and neck?

Balance Issues - The cerebellum, which controls your motor stability and maintains equilibrium, is full of GABA receptors and is heavily affected by benzos. When damaged, it can affect your ability to maintain balance. This is often the cause of falls in the elderly. This area of the brain can take a while to be fully restored. Exercises designed to help return equilibrium can aid in recovery.

Dizziness/Lightheadedness/Vertigo - Along with anticholinergics and antihistamines, benzodiazepines are commonly used as vestibular suppressants and are often taken by people who suffer from motion sickness, motion sensitivity, and vertigo. When the drugs are removed, your vestibular system reacts and can cause dizziness and lightheadedness during recovery.

Headache/Migraines - Headaches are another common complaint during withdrawal and are often combined with pressure in the forehead and temples. Some complain that it feels like there is a tight band around their head. Migraines can also be triggered during this time.

Neck Pain - Neck pain often occurs in conjunction with headaches and sometimes chest pain. This is most likely due to muscle tightness in the area, which is aggravated by stress and the reduction of the benzodiazepines — benzos are excellent muscle relaxants.

Slurred Speech - Dysarthria is the medical term for difficulty speaking, which is indicated by slow or slurred speech. It's often a result of neurological injury, which can include benzodiazepine dependence and withdrawal. This can be exacerbated by alcohol and lack of sleep.

Throat Tightening - In addition to difficulty swallowing, some people also feel like their throat is tightening or swollen. This is a common symptom of excessive anxiety, so it's no surprise that it also appears during withdrawal. Relaxation exercises can help ease the tension in the neck.

Did you experience balance issues or dizziness?

I have suffered from frequent vertigo and light-headedness during my twelve years on Klonopin, but I always attributed that to an earlier inner-ear issue. Allow me to explain.

Years ago, before my experience with benzos, I had an inner ear infection from a cold. I got dizzy, so I took a Scopolamine Transdermal Patch that I had for an upcoming trip to treat motion sickness. It helped, but anytime I tried to stop using the patch I got violently sick. Room spinning, vomiting, all the fun stuff.

Over a period of five months, I went to a variety of specialists who suggested everything from bizarre viruses to a brain tumor. Eventually, I saw the top otologist in the Kansas City area — which is where I was living at the time — and he diagnosed me in ten minutes. It appears I had inner ear damage from the cold virus, which is not uncommon, but that the Scopolamine patch prevented my brain from adjusting to the injury so I couldn't regain my equilibrium. Anyway, he told me to taper off the patch slowly, which I did, and I recovered.

Unfortunately, it didn't end there. I would still get dizzy and had bouts of periodic vertigo. When this happened, I would just have to stop everything, lie down, and wait for it to pass. These episodes lasted for many years and started at the same time I began taking clonazepam. For over a decade, I attributed my ongoing vertigo to my inner ear damage, but I'm not so sure anymore. When I read about vertigo, light-headedness, and dizziness being possible symptoms of benzos, it made me re-evaluate the cause. You see, my vertigo has nearly disappeared since I have withdrawn from benzos.

So, was I in tolerance during that time and vertigo was just an early symptom? Or am I attributing too many common biological maladies to benzos unfairly? I'll probably never know for sure.

Did you have other head and neck issues?

I have experienced headaches, neck pain, and throat tightening during withdrawal. Are all these attributed to benzo withdrawal? I don't really know, but I think most of them have something to do with it. The throat tightening happened very early on in my withdrawal, perhaps one of the first symptoms I had. It went together with difficulty swallowing. I could always breathe, and it was more annoying than scary.

I also struggled with chronic neck and shoulder tightness. As I mentioned, I carry my stress in my neck/shoulders and in my pelvic area. I can speak more about that in the section on muscular symptoms.

How about migraines?

As far as I can recall, I had never experienced a migraine before withdrawal. My wife has them periodically and has shared the experience with me. Throbbing pain, extreme sensitivity, visual disturbances — not something I am eager to try. I am grateful that I do not suffer from migraines. But then, just the other day, something strange happened.

I returned to working on my book after lunch, and I was having some trouble with my vision. It was weird. I couldn't see the screen right in front of me. There were these crystalline, computer-like images floating in my view. I've had floaters in my vision before, like something on the surface of my eye, but this was different. I'd never experienced this. No matter what I tried to do, I couldn't read the words on the screen. I was tired because I'd been writing since five that morning, so I laid down for about 10 minutes. But no change. In fact, when I closed my eyes, the images would not go away.

Then I remembered something about vision and migraines, and I asked my wife about it. She said that my symptoms sounded like a migraine to her. She gave me a Pepsi and some ibuprofen, her home remedy, and told me to lay down in a dark, quiet room. I followed her instructions, and after about 40 minutes it went away. I never had the extreme head pain that is common, but my wife said that sometimes a migraine can be just visual. That is the only one I have experienced so far, and I hope it stays that way.

As with so many symptoms I have listed here, I can't say that withdrawal was the cause — or partial cause — of my migraine. It might have just been stress and lack of sleep. I'll probably never know. All I do know is that had never happened to me before.

How about slurred speech?

Just like the vertigo, I had several symptoms during tolerance that I attributed to other factors since I was unaware of the issues with benzos at the time. One of these was slurred speech.

About five or so years ago, I was quite involved in the film industry. I was on the advisory board of one film festival and taught screenwriting at several others. During most of these events, I got little sleep and drank more alcohol than usual. It was during these events that I noticed I would start to slur my speech, especially when I'd been drinking. If I slowed down my pace of speech, I could usually get my words out, but it was difficult at best.

At the time, I attributed it to drinking alcohol, combined with lack of sleep. But the strange thing was, I never had this problem before — even in college when my drinking was far more frequent. If I had researched the medication I was taking, I may have discovered that this was a tolerance symptom of benzos. But I never investigated it.

My slurring of speech has eased a bit, although I still experience it when I'm exhausted. I'm just glad that I know the cause now.

Symptoms of the Heart & Lungs

So, moving on to the heart and lungs. What are the symptoms here?

Typical types of heart and lung symptoms include the following:

Breathing Difficulties - As I discussed in "Benzo Usage," breathing difficulties are common including hyperventilation (over-breathing) and hypoventilation (depressed breathing). Benzos can suppress respiration and have a track record of affecting breathing patterns. When mixed with opiates, they can cease breathing altogether causing death. If you feel you have significant breathing issues during withdrawal, please speak with your doctor immediately.

Flushing/Sweating/Skin Conditions - Flushing, excessive sweating, burning of the skin, heat rashes, and related skin conditions are part of the benzodiazepine hall-of-crazy-symptoms. They can be quite irritating and occasionally painful, but they're rarely dangerous.

Heart Palpitations - Heart palpitations are another one of the scary symptoms that often send people to the emergency room. These are also common in panic attacks and heightened states of anxiety but are usually benign. Beta blockers help some people during withdrawal if the palpitations are severe. Consult with your doctor if you feel these are needed.

And your experience?

I had all three of these. You guessed that though, didn't you?

I had constant flushing early on during withdrawal. Mostly at night when I tried to sleep. I now have a lot more sympathy toward women who go through menopause. Red bumps still cover my chest and sides. My dermatologist told me they're benign, so I don't worry too much about them now. Periodic heart palpitations were fun. I often thought I was having a heart attack, either because of heart palpitations or chest pain. The palpitations have since subsided, and my experience with them lasted only a few months.

Breathing is the odd one, though. And a terrifying one at that. When I was sleeping, there were times I'd suddenly wake up gasping for breath. There were also many times when I was meditating that I calmed down so much and then suddenly needed to find my breath again. It was distressing at first, but I became accustomed to it over time.

While these symptoms are common, it's a good idea to get them checked out by a doctor.

Muscular Symptoms

Why do our muscles seem to be so affected by withdrawal?

Benzos are very effective muscle relaxants. By the time the drugs are removed from your system the muscles have been chemically re-laxed for months or even years, and now they need to figure out how to behave in this new drug-free environment. The removal of a long-term muscle relaxant, in addition to damage to the nerves that signal the muscles, can create a painful cascade effect with some bizarre results. Even the headaches I mentioned earlier might be partly attributed to muscle tension. Muscular symptoms during withdrawal can include aches, convulsions, fatigue, jerks, pains, pulls, spasms, sprains, stiffness, tears, tics, tremors, twitches, and overall weakness. Sounds like fun, doesn't it?

The good news is that none of these are harmful in the long-term. The bad news is that you must deal with them in the short-term. Exercise is critical to a healthy recovery, but chronic muscle stiffness can make that difficult at times. I had several pulls and sprains during my tenure with withdrawal in my legs, arms, and chest. This included recurring costochondritis, which is inflammation of the cartilage that joins your rib muscles to the breastbone. That's a particularly fun one since it can feel like you're having another heart attack. And so, another trip to the emergency room. Physical therapy helped me recover from this one by doing very limited stretching exercises.

Muscle pain was also quite common. Random pains throughout the body with little or no cause. I still get these a lot. I did have minor convulsions, shaking, and tremors now and then, but usually only when my anxiety was extremely high.

What about paralysis or seizures?

Since benzodiazepines are sometimes prescribed as an anti-seizure medication, it follows that withdrawal can cause seizures in some people. This is most common in patients who withdraw too quickly and rare in those who taper slowly. Convulsions can accompany seizures or occur independently. Temporary paralysis is also possible.

These are the extremes of the benzo symptomology spectrum. Few symptoms are as terrifying or dangerous. Please seek medical help immediately if you experience these symptoms.

What can we do to help ease these muscle issues?

Most of the muscle issues can be handled by moderate stretching and limiting movement. Avoid any strenuous workouts without proper stretching before and after. The main thing is to listen to your body. Exercise if you can, but don't push it too hard. Your body is recovering, and you need to let it. Be kind to your muscles. But being sedentary should only be a short-term solution. When you can get up and move, do so, just take it slowly.

Nerve Sensations

What type of nerve sensations are you referring to?

I touched on a few of these earlier, like akathisia (inner trembling and restless), burning sensation of the skin, muscle tics, tremors, and spasms, but there are others like electric shocks, hypersensitivity, itching, paresthesia, and skin rashes. The good news is that these symptoms, although annoying and sometimes painful, are not permanent. They recede along with the rest of the symptoms during withdrawal, although it might take a while.

I've heard of paresthesia and formication. What are these?

Paresthesia refers to strange sensations on or near the surface of the skin with no apparent physical cause. Common complaints include burning, tingling, pins and needles, numbness, or even electrical impulses. Formication is a unique type of paresthesia usually identified by the feeling of something crawling on the skin, like a spider or bug.

And let me guess, you had this too?

This is one of my more persistent symptoms. My version usually takes the form of spiders crawling on my face, most often on the left side near the temple. Sometimes I press my hand on my face or wrap a towel around my head, just to keep pressure on the area to ease the sensation. The spiders were very distressing when it first started happening, but much like the tinnitus, I have learned to accept it over time.

Immune & Endocrine Symptoms

What about the immune system? And the endocrine system?

Some people seem to get more infections during withdrawal. This one is anecdotal and hard to prove or disprove, not that the others are any easier in that realm. Since most of us are under more stress during withdrawal, and we know that chronic stress can lower our immune system's ability to fight off germs, this makes sense. Depression also can be a cause of diminished immunity.

Another factor is that people going through withdrawal might be living a less healthy lifestyle. Many can't exercise due to muscle tightness, body pain, or social phobias. Others have a limited diet and aren't getting the nutrition that they need. Keeping a healthy lifestyle can be a struggle, but it's a struggle that is worth fighting. We need to keep ourselves as healthy as we can now more than ever.

As for the endocrine system, we know that benzos have an effect, but there is little information on this topic from related studies. Some women complain about menstrual difficulties, but these are common in the general population too, so it's hard to determine a cause and effect. Both male and female patients have occasionally complained about breast swelling and engorgement during withdrawal. The good news is that most endocrine system issues do improve once withdrawal is complete.

And yes, before you even ask, I did struggle with some immune system issues during withdrawal, but luckily not endocrine issues that I can identify.

Okay, then. Is that it for the list of symptoms?

As far as this book is concerned, yes. But that doesn't mean that there aren't other symptoms that could be attributed to benzos. I just wanted to discuss the most common ones.

CHAPTER 13

MANAGING THE FEAR

What is the number one enemy to a successful withdrawal?

That's easy. Fear.

Can you elaborate?

Sure.

In my opinion, fear, and the stress and anxiety related to that fear, cause more distress and more complications during withdrawal than anything else. Fear that we're drug dependent. Fear that we're drug addicted. Fear of this symptom, or that one. Fear that this symptom is a sign of a heart attack. Fear that this one is cancer. Or that this one is MS or Parkinson's or Alzheimer's. Fear that this one will be permanent. Fear that we won't be able to work or find another job. Fear that our relationships won't survive the stress. Fear that we will lose our homes. Fear that we will be locked up in a mental institution. And at the end of it all, fear that we won't be able to cope with life without the help of those damn benzos that created the whole problem in the first place.

And this fear is not some natural psychological fear. It's chemically enhanced. On top of the original anxieties we had before our dependence on benzos, we now have a damaged nervous system that can't process fear correctly. A system that can send us into a panic state — both psychologically and physiologically — at the least sign of distress.

> *Many "withdrawal symptoms" are simply due to fear of withdrawal (or even fear of that fear). People who have had bad experiences have usually been withdrawn too quickly (often by doctors!) and without any explanation of the symptoms.*[347]

— Prof. Ashton

But how do we deal with the fear that those of us with anxiety have been battling for years?

There's no overnight fix. As much as we all want one, it just doesn't exist. But there are a lot of things we can do to manage this fear and develop a more positive and stable mindset.

Like many of us, you may have physical symptoms. But rarely can you do anything to directly affect them. They will come, and they will go. And often, those physical symptoms are triggered or aggravated by your mental state. Fear, stress, and anxiety play a significant role in determining the severity of withdrawal. Therefore, it just makes sense for us to spend more time and effort on managing our fear and anxiety and less on trying to figure out how to physically mitigate each individual symptom.

Can you define this mindset you're talking about?

I was blind-sided by intense fear when I first learned about the horrors of withdrawal. This fear crippled me more times than I care to remember. Benzo withdrawal is a significant life experience. The fear of the pain, discomfort, life changes, and everything else that may come with it is natural and expected. But, most of the time our fears are far worse than the actual process of withdrawal.

> *Many people are frightened of withdrawal, but reports of having to "go through hell" can be greatly exaggerated.*[348]

— Prof. Ashton

I feared that I wouldn't have the strength to taper and become benzo-free. I was afraid that I would be on the drugs the rest of my life. I was worried I would have attacks and that I would lose my home and my wife. But none of that happened. Yes, I'm four years off benzos, and I still have symptoms. But guess what? I did it. I am benzo-free. And many of my fears never came true.

A proper mindset is all about managing the fear and reducing the worry. Less worry = less anxiety = less symptoms. That's the plan.

> *Above all, stop worrying. Worry, fear and anxiety increase all withdrawal symptoms. Many of these symptoms are actually due to anxiety and not signs of brain or nervous system damage. People who fear withdrawal have more intense symptoms than those who just take it as it comes and think positively and confidently about recovery.*[349]

— Prof. Ashton

But you still worried, didn't you?

Hell, yes. I would have a Ph.D. in worry, if there were such a thing. I learned this great skill from my family. In my family, worry is normal. It's expected. The right to worry is often defended. Crazy, isn't it?

On top of that, I'm ADHD and recovering from benzos, so now my over-thinking is amplified. I can't turn my mind off, and I rarely can steer it where I want it to go. It just takes off in any which way, and I have to catch up to it and see what it's been up to. If my mind always chose happy places to go, that wouldn't be so bad; but too often my mind chooses dark, depressing, and even angry places. Oh, the joy.

I've done my best to break the cycle of worry over the years, with some success here and there. But when I learned of my dependence on benzos, well, it came rushing back like the Great Flood. I know objectively that 99% of all worry is useless, and yet I couldn't stop. Quite often I would obsess on some negative thought for five or ten minutes before I even know I started. I wish to hell that I could find the remote control to my own brain so I could turn it off, or at least hit pause every now and then.

I'm a worrier too. It's what I do.

And that statement may be part of our problem.

Celeste, one of the three counselors I visited during withdrawal, helped me understand my addiction to worry. She put it into words that really spoke to me. I would often say to her in a session that "I'm a worrier" or that "I have anxiety" or that "my brain is just wired wrong." She didn't like that type of self-talk, and for a good reason. I was just re-enforcing a negative stereotype of myself. Instead, she taught me to say the following:

I have a habit and pattern of fear and scaring myself.

This helped. It really did. Instead of looking at it as a life sentence of weakness, I saw my worrying as a habit. And habits can be changed. I still have a lot of work to do, but I am making progress. Thanks to Celeste for her sage advice.

I survived benzo withdrawal, even with that crazy over-reactive brain of mine. I did it through hard work and with a great deal of help from a lot of different people. I finally found a positive mindset for withdrawal, and I think you can too.

Okay, I'm with you. So, what do I do?

The first step to finding a positive mindset for withdrawal is realizing that fear — and obsessing about that fear — makes your symptoms worse. It makes your withdrawal harder. Recognizing and accepting that is a huge first step. I'm not saying that fear is always the enemy. Fear is a useful emotion in certain circumstances, especially when triggered by outside influences. And accepting that fear is critical to processing that emotion. The problem comes when we ruminate.

Ruminating literally means to "chew the cud." This description works great for cows but might not be so palatable for humans. In psychology, ruminating usually means to focus on one's distress and its causes rather than on its solutions. In the benzo world, you will find a disproportionate percentage of people who excel in this technique. We know how to ruminate. And it gets us into a lot of trouble.

Learning how to accept the fear but reduce the rumination is the real goal here. I found five key areas where I improved on my ability to manage my anxiety. They are responsibility, positivity, activity, kindness, and acceptance. I'll touch on each one here just to help you understand my thinking.

Responsibility for what?

Your own health and recovery.

Usually the best judge is you, yourself; you must be in control and must proceed at the pace that is comfortable for you.[350]

— Prof. Ashton

For many of us who have developed benzodiazepine dependence, this condition is an iatrogenic illness — an illness caused by a medical procedure or treatment. That was true in my case and in so many others. My doctor prescribed benzos for my ongoing stomach distress, and I took the drug for the following twelve and a half years. The first eleven of those years, I switched doctors a few times, but they each continued my prescription without voicing any concern. Was I mad about that? Of course, I was. I was furious.

But, eventually, I started looking at myself and at my role in this whole thing. In all that time, I never really thought about the drug I was taking. I just took it. I could have looked it up on the Internet or even asked one of my new docs about any possible complications. But I didn't. I just trusted that my doctors knew best. Why didn't I ask? Why didn't I look it up? Perhaps I didn't want to know. Maybe it just didn't occur to me. I can't say for sure.

Regardless of how small my part was in this whole fiasco, I did play a role. Even if it was just one percent. Learning that, noticing that, taught me a precious lesson: I am responsible for my health. No one else. It's my brain, my body, and I'm in charge. I now approach my relationships with medical professionals as that of a partnership. Sure, my doctor knows a lot more about medicine than I ever will. But she doesn't know everything. And neither does the Internet. While it can be an excellent resource for some medical information, it's also full of inaccuracies, hype, and biased personal accounts. Common sense is critical.

I learned to be a partner with my doctor, instead of a submissive patient. I now have a say in what happens to me. If I don't like a prescription, I may get a second opinion. Or a third. I may even suggest an alternative. I decide what is done to my body, and nobody else. I'll never take another prescribed medication without doing my own thorough research. I'll never go through another medical procedure without fully understanding all the risks and weighing the pros and cons.

Once I realized that I was in charge, I also knew that I couldn't do this alone. Dr. V was on board, so that was half the battle. Along the way, I added a massage therapist, a physical therapist, a few counselors, some medical specialists, and other support personnel to my team. To round things out, I had an incredibly loving and supportive wife and a fantastic family to back me up. I had a formidable team. One that I relied on often.

Taking responsibility means taking the lead in your recovery. You're in charge, and that's a good thing.

What about positivity? And if you're going to say, "just be positive," I might have to kill you.

Well, then I won't do that. Let me take a different approach.

Allowing your feelings to happen, all feelings, is critical to maintaining mental health. A positive mindset is not about suppressing your feelings or glossing over them and putting on a good face. That plan of attack can lead to disaster. What I'm talking about is a positive mindset. You still feel sad, angry, mad, and everything else at different times. But when something happens in your life, you will lean a bit more on the positive side than the negative side. Focus on what is good in your life. That's all it is. The glass is half-full.

Argue for your limitations, and sure enough they're yours.[351]

— Richard Bach, *Illusions*

It's estimated that we have about 50,000 thoughts in the average day. That's a lot. And many of these thoughts — perhaps even most of them — are distorted. Our senses perceive the outside world, but those messages go through a filter of habits, patterns, opinions, ideas, and stories before creating a final thought or emotion.

One of the best methods for changing your way of thinking is to learn to recognize negative thought patterns. Something psychologists call cognitive distortions. These include techniques, such as mind-reading, labeling, emotional reasoning, blaming, fortune-telling, personalization, catastrophizing (one of my personal favorites), and several others. As a chronic over-thinker, I'm guilty of every one of these distortions at one time or another. And I'm not alone.

Another method is to remember to enjoy life, despite your current situation. I thought I would be fully recovered a long time ago, but I'm not. And it's possible that I may never be. So, should I wait until I am fully recovered to start enjoying life again? I don't think so. I need to enjoy it along the way. Celebrate the journey, not just the end game. The real joy is in getting there. That is the guts of life.

Let me use an example here. As I'm writing this section, Stephen Hawking passed away. What a loss. Here is a person who was diagnosed with ALS in 1963 and given only a few years to live. Not only did he live for another 55 years, well into his seventies, but he thrived and became one of the greatest scientific minds of our time. He took a terribly debilitating disease and lived a full and productive life.

> *My advice to other disabled people would be, concentrate on things your disability doesn't prevent you doing well, and don't regret the things it interferes with. Don't be disabled in spirit as well as physically.*[352]

— Stephen Hawking

Noticing these patterns in yourself and working to change them is a significant first step towards reducing the worry and anxiety. Once you've identified them, you can start to change them.

But everything in the world is so negative these days. How do you find something good to focus on?

I know. War, terrorism, school-shootings, obesity, health care, eroding freedoms, cancer, climate change, and on and on. Life is so much worse now — isn't it?

Let's take a quick look:

- In the 1300s, the bubonic plague wiped out one-third of the entire human race. Today, we have either eradicated or significantly reduced the effects of polio, smallpox, tuberculosis, cholera, the Spanish flu, and the bubonic plague.
- In 1800, 88% of the world population was illiterate. In 2014, that number was less than 15%.[353]
- From 1981 to 2013, the global population living in absolute poverty dropped from 44% to less than 11%.[354]
- From 1994 to 2014, the number of U.S. victims of violent crime per capita decreased by a whopping 75%.[355] And yet, most people believe crime is actually getting worse.[356]
- Today, many of us have access to air-conditioning, airplanes, automobiles, dishwashers, electricity, indoor plumbing, the Internet, lawn mowers, microwave ovens, paved roads, radio, TV, video games, and so many other labor-saving, time-saving, life-saving, and pleasure-inducing inventions.

There are a hundred more stats that I would love to share, but I think I made my point.

We worry so much about how bad the world has become when, by most measurements, the exact opposite is true. These are incredibly positive trends. The world is a better place to live now than almost any time in history. I understand that if you're in the middle of benzo withdrawal that life might suck. Big time. I can't argue that one. But if you can find a little bit of good news to hang on to every now and then, it can make the process a little bit easier.

And what about activity? Do you mean mind or body?

Both. We touched on this a bit in chapter 12, but let's get into a bit more detail here.

More and more studies show that keeping your mind active is key to keeping it healthy. This goes double for people with anxiety and triple for people going through benzo withdrawal. If you're currently working, keep working. Don't quit unless you need to. If you aren't working, find something to keep you busy. Learn something. Take an online class. Read books. Volunteer. Prove the theory of cold fusion and solve world hunger. Write a book.

There may be days when you feel you can't do anything, and that's okay. But when you can, do so. Don't lay there in bed and contemplate the sad state of your life. I've done that, and it ain't no fun. When you don't feel like getting up, try anyway.

Throughout much of my taper and early withdrawal, I had a voice in the back of my head. It was that of a fish. Dory, from the Pixar movie *Finding Nemo*. "Just keep swimming. Just keep swimming. Just keep swimming..."[357] It became a sort of mantra of mine. Keeping your mind busy is one of the great secrets to managing benzo withdrawal. I occupied my mind with research. Research on benzos. On happiness. On psychology. On anxiety and insomnia and alternative treatments. And all of that became the basis for this book. A win-win scenario if I've ever seen one.

And being physically active is equally as important.

A 2000 research study evaluated three groups of patients who treated their major depression with medication (sertraline), exercise, or a combination of the two. Although all three groups showed similar improvement early on, when tested six months later, the results were startling. The medication-only group had a 38% relapse rate, the combination group had a 31% relapse rate, and the exercise only group had just a 9% relapse rate.[358]

And it doesn't take much. Studies have shown that the first twenty minutes of exercise garners the most health benefits. Even if you can't do anything else, a brisk walk every day can do wonders. It's not just about exercise, it's about being active. "Just keep swimming."

Regular to moderate exercise is recommended during with-drawal...The aim is to lead a healthy lifestyle which by definition in-cludes some exercise in a form that is enjoyable for you.[359]

— Prof. Ashton

Why kindness? Be kind to who?

Everyone. Friends. Enemies. Family. Strangers. Yourself. Especially yourself.

It all starts at home. Be kind to yourself. I learned to not judge myself so harshly. If I messed up during withdrawal, that's okay. I'll make mistakes, and I'll be okay. I learned to let it go and move on. I needed to take care of myself first, especially during this time. I set boundaries and let those who love me know what they were. I found quiet time whenever I could to allow my body and mind to heal. I treated myself to small pleasures to help raise my spirits and my self-esteem. If I ever needed to be kind to myself, this was the time.

I also had to remember to be kind to those around me. Most people don't really understand what we're going through. How can they? So, help them. Realize that this is hard for them too. It's frustrating when people don't understand the scope of your illness. But how can anyone genuinely understand this who hasn't experienced it? It's like me telling a PTSD-plagued Vietnam vet that I understand what he went through. I can try. I can even watch all the movies and read all the books about that time. I can research the ongoing struggles of veterans after they come home. But I'll never truly understand what it was like.

So, help those around you understand what it's like for you. Help them find patience with you in this trying time. Help them realize that you're doing everything in your power to get better. Realize that they will never fully understand this experience you're going through but accept what love and support they can provide without judgment. They may doubt your symptoms, they may question that you're even sick, and that's okay. Help them help you.

And what about acceptance?

One of the best things that happened to me during withdrawal was when I found acceptance. I stopped struggling and fighting my symptoms and instead accepted my current condition. Acceptance can be a difficult pill to swallow for many people (no pun intended). It sounds easy, but it's a difficult transition and it usually only comes with time.

Most people experiencing benzo withdrawal see their recovery as a struggle. A fight. A battle of epic proportions. And it can be. They want to do everything they can to make it disappear. And if they can't make it go away, then make it as easy as possible. Find a way to have fewer symptoms. Or make it be over sooner. They want to find a shortcut. They want to find some substance or elixir that will make things all better.

I had this same attitude for most of my withdrawal. I fought it. Every time I had a new symptom, I wanted to know why. What caused this one? What can I do to make it go away? How long will it last? Why is my body doing this? Why is this happening to me? What can I do to stop it? The precious few answers seemed to vary from day to day. And while I received a lot of support, there were never any real solutions.

Over time, this pattern got old. I started to see the futility of it. My symptoms continued regardless of what I did. And eventually, my attitude towards them slowly changed. I began to find acceptance. I learned to back off and let my body do what it's been trying to do all along.

And what was that?

Heal.

That's all that benzo withdrawal really is; it's your body healing. And healing is a good thing. In fact, it's an amazing thing. Our bodies heal even from some of the most horrendous injuries. It's an incredible piece of biochemical engineering. And the best thing I could do was let it do its job.

Once I accepted that I was dependent on benzos and that all this mess was just my body healing, my whole attitude started to change. Sure, I still get symptoms, but they don't bother me as much. In fact, they rarely make me anxious anymore. And if they aren't making me anxious, then the cycle is broken, or at least fractured. Less anxiety equals less symptoms. I'm benzo-free now, so the benzos are out of my system, and they're not damaging my GABA receptors anymore. All that's left is me and my body, and my body wants time to heal.

Now, this healing process is painful at times. And there are times of struggle. But, there's also a reason for it all. It makes sense. That makes it bearable. We're talking about nerves here. The messengers of pain. So, I really have two choices: I can fight this process, which really means I'm competing against my own body's attempt to heal itself. Or, I can allow the healing to take place and try and live with the discomfort as best I can throughout the process.

Perfect timing. Just as I'm writing this, my left thumb has started to twitch uncontrollably. I'm not kidding nor making this up for effect. I've been going through a mild wave lately, so it's not a big surprise. I could obsess about my thumb and try and make it stop. I could ruminate and look on the boards to see if anyone still has muscle twitches in protracted withdrawal. I could start to worry that I have MS or Parkinson's. But none of that would really help. It doesn't work that way. I'm sure my thumb is a little tired from typing today and that combined with my recent wave of symptoms — well, it all makes sense. So, I tell myself it's healing, and I think the best thing is to step away from the computer and take a break. I'll let my thumb rest and do something else for a while.

In fact, I think I'll go take a nap. Yes, I take naps in the middle of the afternoon. I'm out of work and spending most of my time writing this book. I've found that taking a brief break in the middle of the day to allow my system to calm down and rest helps my recovery. So, that's what I do. I'll be back in a bit.

***** INTERMISSION *****
(cue elevator music)

Okay, I'm back. I see you got some popcorn.

I was hungry. Are you better now?

Yes, thank you. Hope you didn't miss me too much.

Still twitching?

The twitching lasted for about 30 minutes. Not too unusual. It wasn't painful. More annoying than anything else. I decided not to fight it, and I even got a brief nap in on top of it. I'm doing just fine now. Back to the topic at hand.

Acceptance is not about surrender, giving up, or anything like that. It's not about letting others push me around. It's about accepting life as it is and not fighting against it at every turn. It's about living in balance — living in harmony with my body and the world around me. I take care of myself and manage my symptoms in a healthy way. I realize that this journey with benzos happened to me. It's in the past. It doesn't matter if it was someone else's fault or my own. All that matters is that it happened, it's part of my life now, and I have to figure out how to live with it.

Suffering and struggle are parts of life. Important parts. They carry with them some fantastic gifts if only we look for them. Benzo withdrawal brought some fantastic gifts to me. I'm not saying I want to do it all over again, not by a long shot. Instead, I'm looking past the pain and finding the change that has been created in me. That includes a very positive change in my attitude and how I approach my life. A change that I don't believe I would have found without this experience.

Life is full of ups and downs. I have a damaged nervous system now. It's a fact. I hope it gets better over time, but it might not. And you know what? That's okay. I'm much better than I was in the middle of withdrawal, and I am grateful for that. In fact, I appreciate life so much more now because of what I went through. I'm a better person now, and that's kinda cool.

Anything else?

That's it for managing the fear. Let's move onto setting boundaries.

CHAPTER 14

SETTING BOUNDARIES

What do you mean by boundaries?

One of the most consistent rules that I have discovered in every facet of my life is that of balance. It holds true in 98.652% of all situations (yes, I made that number up). For most people, life is rarely lived in the extremes. Most of us live it somewhere in the middle. And that makes a lot of sense. Unfortunately, during withdrawal, that balance is a bit tougher to maintain. So, we adjust. And we set boundaries to help us get through this challenging time.

What boundaries are you talking about?

Boundaries during withdrawal come in a wide variety of shapes and sizes. Some of them relate to diet. Others relate to exercise or entertainment. Some even apply to relationships with other people. Overall, boundaries are limitations we place on our lives to help us reduce adverse reactions and to help manage our recovery. But setting boundaries isn't always straightforward. It's easy to make your boundaries too restrictive or have them adversely affect those around you.

One of the most common themes throughout this book is that

when you go through benzo withdrawal, you have a lot of questions. And this holds true when it comes to setting boundaries. Can I eat sugar? Carbs? Meat? Can I drink caffeine? What about alcohol? Can I smoke weed or cigarettes? Can I take vitamins? How about my herbal supplements? Can I still take benzos under certain circumstances? Should I exercise? Should I improve my relationships or cut the toxic ones? Should I work or stay home and rest? Should I force myself to go outside even for 10 minutes? You get the picture.

These are all great questions, and the answers will vary dramatically depending on whom you ask. I've identified two distinct schools of thought on boundaries during withdrawal:

Avoidance - Most people on the online benzo boards fall into the "avoidance" camp. The argument made here is that benzo withdrawal is already so arduous for some people, why would you do anything that might make it worse? This is a valid argument and is based on solid, common-sense principles. It just makes sense that if something is making you feel worse, avoid it, especially during this difficult time.

Lifestyle - The second school of thought is what I like to call "lifestyle." It takes a more laid-back approach to boundaries, focusing more on maintaining some sense of normalcy during withdrawal. This is more closely aligned with Prof. Ashton's thoughts and reasoning from her manual:

> *Some people advise that caffeine and alcohol should be completely ruled out. However, the point about gradual dosage tapering at home is that people should get used to living a normal lifestyle without drugs.*[360]

So, which school of thought do you subscribe to?

I believe there needs to be a balance here. Big surprise, huh?

Some of the subjects on the boards garner more agreement from within the community, others more dissension. Some people apparently have an issue to promote for one reason or the other and will try to convince you that their way is the right way. Some believe that a particular substance is the root of all evil. Others may tell you that that same substance saved their lives. Some people cut people out of their lives who don't understand them or what they're going through. Others cling tighter to the people in their lives despite their attitudes. Some people stay at home and never leave. Others challenge withdrawal at every turn and force themselves to live some semblance of a normal life. It's incredibly confusing to know whom to listen to and whom to ignore.

Let's look at diet for a minute. Prof. Ashton says, "In my opinion there is no need to be over-obsessive about diet."[361] The anxiety generated around being hyper-vigilant about every substance you put into your body can cause as much damage, if not more, as the substance itself. I see it all the time. But then you speak to someone with severe benzo belly who can't eat so much as a piece of bread without a severe reaction, and you quickly realize that avoidance makes a lot of sense too. Why would you do, eat, or drink something that might make you feel worse or delay your healing?

I like moderation. I like balance. Sure, there are a few things that everyone should avoid during withdrawal. But only a few. As for the rest, it will be more trial and error than anything else. Use your own brain to decide for yourself. Try to be as objective as you can in determining what is working for you and what sends you into a wave. And make sure you consider your anxiety and stress levels as factors for your analysis. This can be difficult at times, but it's the only way to really know if something aggravates your symptoms or calms them down.

What boundaries did you set?

All kinds. Relationships was an early one.

I couldn't meet all my family obligations during withdrawal, so I had to tell people "no" quite frequently. As a people-pleaser, that was hard. At first, I would make up excuses why I couldn't leave the house, but eventually, I would be honest and share my condition with them. Some understood, some didn't. But for the most part, I was pleasantly surprised by the support I received.

Getting together with friends or being out in public was a no-go for a long time too. I just couldn't handle the anxiety. I wasn't always sure what to say, or I was afraid that my symptoms would act up and I would be trapped in an awkward or embarrassing situation. If I entered into a heated discussion or debate and got worked up, I would start to shake uncontrollably and had trouble speaking intelligibly. That was a lot of fun. I became cautious with to whom I spoke, what I read, watched, listened to, etc.

News and most media were another problem. The average person lives about 28,000 days on this planet. Most of those days, we wake up and our family is still here, our home is still here, we still have food on the table, entertainment, school, work, trees, air to breathe, water to drink, and so much more. And yet, most of the news and social media hype is about how bad we have it. It's sensational and panders to the scandal-seeking troll in each of us. It was too much for me and my raw nerves to handle, so I just stopped watching it — and still do. And you know what? I don't miss it.

Still, it's all about balance. I didn't want to get too carried away and create an ever-shrinking bubble for myself, or worse, drive the people in my life away from me. Instead, I tried to create a comfortable and safe space to allow my body to heal during this trying time. Just remember, someday you are going to want to return to the real world, eat real food, hang out with real people, even occasionally watch the evening news. The smaller your bubble, the more difficult this transition will be.

What about food and drink?

Many of the questions that we have during withdrawal center around food, drink, and other things we may choose to ingest. Some say avoid everything that might possibly cause issues; others might tell you to chill and see what happens. The choice is yours, and you need to determine your boundaries.

Still, there are a couple of substances that the experts advise we all should avoid during benzo use and withdrawal. Opioids are a big one. The concurrent use of opioids and benzodiazepines can cause life-threatening complications. If you're prescribed an opioid during benzo use or withdrawal, please talk with your doctor immediately about your concerns. Quinolones are another. Fluoroquinolone-based antibiotics should also be avoided when taking or withdrawing from benzos due to possible complications.

Alcohol, caffeine, and sugar are other big players when it comes to avoidance during withdrawal, although the subject can be quite controversial. I think it's time to examine each one of these individually. Come along, it will be fun. Or not.

Alcohol

What about alcohol?

I knew you'd pick that one first.

In my experience, alcohol is the most divisive subject on the benzo boards. There are people in the benzo community who believe that alcohol is the worst thing you can ingest during withdrawal, short of more benzos. And they can be quite vocal about their opinion. There are others who believe it's okay. The fact is, some people claim that they can drink alcohol throughout withdrawal with little or no adverse effects, while others say that alcohol is the number one cause of their waves and symptoms.

This controversy is not going to be solved here. Still, I would be remiss if I didn't discuss it a bit and see where the dispute lies. So, despite my better judgment, let's dive in.

What is Ashton's stance on alcohol?

Prof. Ashton says the following in *The Ashton Manual*:

> *A glass or two of wine is perfectly permissible (and even said by some to be advisable for health). Although it is important not to substitute increasing doses of alcohol for decreasing doses of benzodiazepines, there is no need to deny oneself small pleasures. Moderation is the key: there is no call to be puritanical.*[362]

But in *The Ashton Manual* supplement in April 2011, she also says the following:

Note that alcohol acts like benzodiazepines and should be used, if at all, in strict moderation as advised in this manual.[363]

I am not about to assume I can speak for Prof. Ashton here, but it appears from her statements that she believes it is important to live as normal of a life as possible during withdrawal but to be cautious with alcohol since it acts like benzos.

What do others say?

The general agreement from the various online benzo boards is to avoid alcohol throughout withdrawal. Some take an adamant stance against it while others say it generally should be avoided.

> *Alcohol acts on some of the same GABA receptors in the brain as benzodiazepines. Your receptors are already vulnerable from the benzodiazepine withdrawal. It is most likely for this reason that many report alcohol intensifies their withdrawal symptoms.*[364]

— BenzoBuddies

Their point is that you don't want to add another substance into your body that affects the same receptors that are in the process of healing during withdrawal. Since many people in the benzo community have found that alcohol increases the frequency and severity of their symptoms, this makes perfect sense. Some people have suggested that you wait to drink alcohol until after your last dose of benzos, while others say to wait until you're completely symptom-free. Some even say that you should never drink again.

As with almost every aspect of benzo withdrawal, we don't have a lot of facts here. All the evidence is anecdotal and based on each individual's experience and interpretation of what is causing his or her symptoms.

Did you drink during withdrawal?

I was never a heavy drinker before, no more than a couple of beers in a week. So, when it came time for withdrawal, drinking or not drinking wasn't a big issue. I drank very rarely during my taper, but then stopped entirely during acute and most of protracted withdrawal. By the time I took my last dose of clonazepam, I had read post after post about how dangerous alcohol was, and it started to stress me out. I finally decided to stop drinking for a while. Still, I miss the normalcy of it.

What do you mean by "normalcy of it?"

After years of dealing with benzo withdrawal, I desperately wanted some semblance of what I like to call "normalcy." All the things I couldn't do anymore really started to pile up, and I just wanted some sense of a normal life. Going out to dinner with my wife and friends at a neighborhood bar and grill and having a nice pint of lager is a small slice of heaven for me, and I miss it. For the longest time, I couldn't have dessert, I couldn't have caffeine, I couldn't have alcohol. It really started to add up, and it's been quite depressing, especially after five years now.

The only real evidence I can go by is how my body reacts when I have alcohol. Occasionally, I would drink one night as a test just to see if I had a reaction the next day, or the next. I never found any direct correlation. My windows and waves would come and go. The only consistent triggers for my waves have been sugar, stress, and anxiety. Especially the last two. The more stressed I am, or the more anxious I am, the more likely I'll go into a wave. But as far as alcohol goes, I just haven't seen a connection.

I'm now four years off, and I still avoid alcohol most of the time. I might have a beer once every few months or so, but that's it. I still don't drink hard liquor, but that was never my preference anyway, thus avoiding it wasn't too hard. Then again, a margarita does tempt me now and then. On the rocks. Salt on the rim. Mmmmm...

So, what's your take on alcohol and withdrawal?

I believe it's wise to avoid it, especially during taper and acute withdrawal.

I think a lot of the caution around alcohol on the benzo boards is well-intended and a good, general course of action. Why take the chance? There are similarities between benzos and alcohol and their effects on GABA receptors. It seems logical that continuous consumption of alcohol during withdrawal very well might complicate this process.

So, I stick with avoidance on this one.

When can I resume drinking after withdrawal?

If you want to play it safe, then wait until you're symptom-free for a time, perhaps six months or so. But the time frame is up to you. Just don't let the obsession with drinking and not drinking cause more problems than the alcohol itself.

What do you mean by obsession?

The main point I am trying to make here is not to let the anxiety about drinking become more detrimental than the alcohol itself. I sometimes see people worry about mouthwash, creams, and all sorts of substances that may have trace amounts of alcohol in them. Or others who have a drink one night and then freak out about it the next day, even before they have any possible adverse reaction. It's my opinion that this fear and obsession can cause as much harm as the alcohol itself.

If you have a drink or two, don't beat yourself up. If you have a bad reaction to that drink, then don't do it again. But don't get worked up about it. Don't obsess about it. What you decide to do is entirely up to you. Gather information and do your own research. Read this book. Read *The Ashton Manual*. Talk to some people online. Make up your own mind.

One thing to remember through all of this is, if you choose to drink, please drink in moderation. Don't let alcohol fill the void left by benzos. And if you have a problem with alcohol, then stay away from it. But you probably already knew that.

Caffeine

What about caffeine?

We can have the same discussion here as we did with alcohol, although perhaps a bit less heated.

> *In my experience, coffee or tea in moderation (about two cups a day), or reasonable amounts of cocoa, chocolate or coca cola, are perfectly compatible with benzodiazepine withdrawal — except in the few individuals who are exquisitely sensitive to caffeine or those with very high anxiety levels.*[365]

— Prof. Ashton

Caffeine is a stimulant. When your body is already overly anxious, then it makes sense that adding a stimulant to the mix might only make matters worse. And that is the case for many people. Especially with those who are struggling with insomnia. The state of hypersensitivity that many of us go through during withdrawal makes us more vulnerable and responsive to the effects of food, drink, and drugs. We can over-respond, and one cup of coffee can feel like we had five.

Did you avoid caffeine?

For the most part, yes.

I started to eat and drink healthier as I was going through withdrawal, as many of us do. For me, it included drinking more tea. Unfortunately, much of the tea you buy at your local coffee shop is caffeinated and it can be a struggle to find decaffeinated tea when you're eating out.

My biggest downfall was Starbucks' Pumpkin Spice Chai. I've been a fan of that drink for years. Unfortunately, it's not very friendly to benzo withdrawal, considering it has its fair share of caffeine and sugar. Still, it was my little treat now and then when I allowed myself. Eventually, I discovered more decaffeinated teas. Especially herbal teas. My current favorite is a hibiscus-based tea blend that I enjoy hot and iced. I also make my own green tea lemonade using decaffeinated green tea and a touch of natural lemon juice.

So yes, I avoided caffeine and still do for the most part. But like I said before, I try not to overthink it. It's not worth the anxiety.

Sugar

What about sugar?

Sugar is one of the big three and perhaps my biggest problem. Even before I started withdrawal, I had cut back on sugar in various ways, including eliminating soda and heavy desserts. Unfortunately, during withdrawal, this wasn't enough. Sugar would really rev me up, and my symptoms would go haywire. I've never been a fan of artificial sweeteners, so that wasn't an option for me. Instead, I slowly reduced my intake of sugar and similar sweeteners throughout my taper and withdrawal.

These days, I almost never eat dessert, except for a small piece of dark chocolate now and then. I drink water at most meals and occasionally decaf tea if it's available. If someone in my party orders a dessert at a restaurant to share, I'll have one or two bites, and I'm satisfied.

Sure, once or twice I have indulged and eaten half a pint of Ben & Jerry's Chunky Monkey ice cream in one sitting. But I always pay for it, and as my symptoms kick in, I know that it was a mistake. Next time I'll just have one bite. It's just not worth the pain.

Other Food & Drink

What other food and drink are of concern?

Some people have problems with MSG, honey, artificial sweeteners, food additives, preservatives, and tasty stuff like that. Many of these are thought to be food sensitivities that people either had prior to withdrawal or developed during the process. Others, like MSG, might have chemical compositions that are specifically difficult for some withdrawing from benzos. But we can take this a bit too far sometimes.

> Advice to cut out white flour, white sugar etc. may help certain individuals but I have also observed that overly restrictive diets can have adverse effects.[366]

— Prof. Ashton

If you're curious about certain substances, I suggest working with a nutritionist who might be able to help you identify a diet that will work best for you. Some people also find that the online benzo boards have useful information about limited diets. Still, I just try to eat a generally healthy diet in moderation. If I find that a specific food is making my symptoms worse, I eliminate it from my diet for a while and see what happens.

Vitamins, Herbs, and Supplements

I take a multivitamin each day. Is this a problem during withdrawal?

This topic is little different from the other ones that I discussed earlier. There are strong opinions on both sides and a few of us — like me again — somewhere in the middle. Many people swear by vitamins, herbs, and supplements. Others believe they do no good and may even be harmful.

> *A normal healthy diet which includes generous amounts of fruit and vegetables and a source of protein and fats (from meat or vegetables), and not too much pure sugar or "junk foods," provides all the nutrients a person needs. There is no general need for dietary supplements or extra vitamins or minerals or for "detoxifying" measures. All these can be harmful in excess.*[367]

— Prof. Ashton

If you eat a healthy diet, you should get enough of the vitamins and minerals that your body needs and won't have a need for supplements. But if you really feel that you're lacking, be careful what you take because it's possible that it might aggravate your withdrawal symptoms.

Are there supplements that I should avoid during withdrawal?

There are no absolutes here, but there are some that you might want to approach with caution. You can always research more details on the benzo boards to learn about others' experiences with them, but just make sure you remember that their experiences will most likely differ from yours. Supplements of concern include chamomile, kava

kava, magnesium, Phenibut, valerian, and vitamins B and D. While these cause problems for some people, others may say that they have found them to be helpful.

I can't say this enough. Although, by now, it sure feels like I have. But, everyone is different. If you believe that a vitamin or herb you're taking is complicating your withdrawal, then stop taking it for a while and see if that helps. If it was prescribed by your physician or another medical professional, then consult with her before you stop. It's a lot of trial and error, and only you can determine what works for you.

Benzos

What about "rescue pills?"

Some patients like to carry a "rescue pill" with them during withdrawal. This is a benzo pill to use in extreme cases when your symptoms and/or anxiety are more than you can handle. While it may provide a sense of security for the patient, it can also lead to updosing, if used. And, this can create more complications during the withdrawal process. If you believe a rescue pill will help you get through withdrawal, please speak with your doctor first.

What about benzos for medical procedures?

Most experts agree that single-dose use of benzos for medical procedures does not complicate withdrawal. This is a relief to those of us who need a way to manage our anxiety during surgery and tests.

> ...a single dose of a benzodiazepine given for an operation does not bring back the addiction.[368]

— Prof. Ashton

> You should not worry that a single dose of a benzodiazepine will cause the reemergence of withdrawal symptoms.[369]

— BenzoBuddies

Still, many of us who have been through withdrawal avoid benzos like the plague. If I can do the procedure without them, that would be my preference. I'm sure I've being overreactive, but can you blame me?

Other Medications

What about other medications?

There are some other drugs, both prescribed and recreational, that can cause complications with benzo use and withdrawal. If you're looking for a medication to help relieve your withdrawal symptoms, then I don't have a lot of good news for you. Most adjuvant medications do little to alleviate withdrawal symptoms and might make things worse. Let's look at a few of these to see what might hurt and what might help.

What about opioids?

Use extreme caution. I think I've already covered this one at length. Please speak with your doctor if you're prescribed opioids while on benzos or in withdrawal. Enough said.

You mentioned fluoroquinolone antibiotics earlier. What's the issue there?

It may be necessary to take antibiotics during benzodiazepine withdrawal but if possible the quinolones should be avoided.[370]

— Prof. Ashton

During benzo use and withdrawal, fluoroquinolones, or quinolones, are best avoided, if possible. The quinolones affect the same GABA receptors as benzodiazepines and can intensify withdrawal symptoms. Familiar brand and generic names of the quinolones include moxifloxacin (Avelox), ciprofloxacin (Cipro), gemifloxacin (Factive), levofloxacin (Levaquin), and ofloxacin.

Even without the complications of benzo use and withdrawal, this class of antibiotics is recommended only in very limited cases. In May of 2016, the FDA revised its boxed warning on quinolones and advised to restrict their use. This warning states that the drugs may cause sudden, severe, and potentially permanent nerve damage, called peripheral neuropathy, along with other complications. In fact, quinolones have GABA antagonistic effects and have been found to displace benzodiazepines from benzodiazepine receptor sites in the body. The announcement also warned about possible side effects, including unusual joint or tendon pain, muscle weakness, a sensation of pins-and-needles on the skin, numbness, confusion, and hallucinations.[371]

Unfortunately, I didn't read — or better yet remember — all the details from *The Ashton Manual* during my withdrawal. And so, when I was prescribed Cipro for an incorrect prostatitis diagnosis, I took it. Why? Because the doctor prescribed it. I know, I should have learned my lesson by then, but I guess I didn't.

As I mentioned earlier, the antibiotic didn't help my condition, which I now believe is related to pelvic floor dysfunction aggravated by benzo withdrawal. Still, now that I know the harmful effects of taking this drug, especially during benzo withdrawal, I wonder if this added to my complications and protracted state. I may never know, but I hope others will learn from my mistakes. And, as you can tell by now, I've made plenty of them to share.

What about antidepressants?

Antidepressants are quite commonly used and can have some benefit. Since suicides have occurred during withdrawal, it may be best to take a more conservative approach to depression treatment during this time. If an SSRI can help prevent suicidal thoughts or severe depressive episodes, it could be well worth it to the patient.

Still, most SSRIs come with their own version of withdrawal. Most will admit it's child's play compared to benzos, but still, it can complicate matters. Look at *The Ashton Manual* for more details about antidepressants during benzo withdrawal, so you have the information you need before speaking with your doctor.

I spoke about my experience with Prozac and Celexa earlier in the book. I tried citalopram (Celexa) before my taper, but I didn't notice a significant benefit to my mood, so I eventually I tapered off the medication. I didn't want another drug that I would have to withdraw from at another time. I was not suicidal at any time, and although I was occasionally depressed, I managed it with counseling and other tools.

Other psych drugs have shown to have little effect to help with withdrawal. This includes antipsychotics, which can aggravate withdrawal.

What about beta blockers?

Beta blockers can be used to help control severe palpitations and muscle tremors. While they have little or no effect on psychological symptoms, they can help relieve the severity of some physical symptoms. Again, like with all medications, you need to consult with your doctor and they should be used only if needed. Beta-blockers should also be tapered slowly if you have taken them for any length of time.

What about sedatives?

I struggled with insomnia, and still do. I hate not sleeping. Lying in bed thinking, which leads to obsessing, which leads to anxiety, which leads to increased withdrawal symptoms, which leads to — you guessed it — insomnia. It's another one of those vicious cycles.

So, I sought help with sleep during withdrawal. My go-to solution was diphenhydramine (Benadryl), as I mentioned earlier. I took this to sleep every night for a few months. It wasn't the best solution, but I was desperate. I knew I couldn't keep it up and I slowly weaned myself off the drugs. I sleep a little better now, and I only use natural tools to aid me in this quest.

Anyway, diphenhydramine is just one of many in the long line of sedatives. Of course, the most common group of sedatives are the z-drugs, or nonbenzodiazepines. Since they behave almost identically to benzodiazepines and have similar withdrawal complications, they're not a recommended option.

Most other hypnotics and sedatives act in a similar way to benzodiazepines, including barbiturates, chloral derivatives (Noctec), ethchlorvynol (Placidyl), zopiclone (Zimovane, Imovane), zolpidem

*(Ambien), zaleplon (Sonata) and, incidentally, alcohol. None of
these drugs should be used as alternative sleeping pills...All can cause
a similar type of dependence and some are more toxic than benzodiazepines.*[372]

— Prof. Ashton

So, where does that leave us? Ashton does mention that tricyclic
antidepressants and some antihistamines can help manage sleep during withdrawal, as I did, but need to be used with caution. No drug is
without side effects.

What about flumazenil?

Now, this is an interesting one.

As I mentioned earlier in this book, there was a study back in 1992
by Lader and Morton that was published in the *Journal of Psychopharmacology*. The study found that patients who received flumazenil in-
fusions had rapid relief of protracted withdrawal symptoms in the
range of 27–82%.[373] Not only did this help prove the existence of benzodiazepine withdrawal syndrome, especially in the protracted state,
but it also alerted doctors to possible medical treatment. It was
thought that flumazenil may help the GABA receptors return to their
natural state after being damaged by long-term benzo use. Wouldn't
that be cool?

Now fast forward to 2018, 25 years later. As you would expect,
benzodiazepine withdrawal syndrome is cured, no one suffers from
abject poverty or hunger, and mermaids and unicorns have mated creating the all too lovable "mermacorn." As if it would be that easy.

There were a few problems with flumazenil in the treatment of
benzodiazepine dependence. First off, the drug must be administered
intravenously and has a very short half-life. As a result, symptom relief is only temporary. Second, it shouldn't be administered to anyone
still taking benzos.[374] So, you must wait until you fully complete your
taper. Oh, and third — just a tiny little thing — treatment with flumazenil comes with a high risk of seizures.

Still, that's not the end of the story for flumazenil. In my research,
I came across detox centers that appear to perform rapid detox from

benzos using flumazenil. In fact, one of them claims they can detox you from benzos in eight days. Personally, I find this highly suspect. It sounds incredible, I'll admit, but I've learned in my experience — especially during my time recovering with benzos — that if it seems too good to be true, it probably is.

Please remember that all the scientific evidence that we have shows that rapid detox from benzos is dangerous and only complicates your withdrawal. After reviewing some patients' experiences with flumazenil, I can't say that it looks very encouraging. With its high risk of seizures and only short-term effectiveness in current studies, I would stick with the standard and proven slow taper if it were me.

What about cannabis?

The use of cannabis is just as controversial as alcohol. While it's still illegal at the federal level in the U.S. and in many other countries, hundreds of people claim that its medicinal benefits are nothing short of life-saving. This includes some people in benzo withdrawal. Of course, there is an equal number of people who say that cannabis has increased their anxiety and made their symptoms worse. Big surprise there, huh?

> *Avoid compensating for benzodiazepines by increasing your intake of alcohol, cannabis or non-prescription drugs.*[375]

— Prof. Ashton

The litany of opinions on benzo recovery and cannabis is almost endless. And, as with most topics in this book, we're not going to solve this issue here. First, though, let's discuss a few facts for those who are curious. There are over a hundred different chemical compounds in cannabis, collectively called cannabinoids. Each one has different properties and can be extracted individually or in combination with other cannabinoids.

Here are three of the most common compounds:

- **THC** (tetrahydrocannabinol) is the primary psychoactive compound responsible for the traditional high that people receive from marijuana.

- **CBD** (cannabidiol) is used most often for medical treatment, including anxiety. It does not have any psychoactive effects when taken alone.
- **CBN** (cannabinol) is also used for medical treatment and as a sleep aid. CBN can be mildly psychoactive since it's derived from the degradation of THC.

Knowing these three types of cannabinoids is important. In regions where cannabis is legal, patients and customers can purchase these cannabinoids in a variety of combinations or individual isolates.

Perhaps the most common compound used in benzo withdrawal is CBD. Many individuals, and some doctors, are touting the benefits of CBD. Since it does not cause the psychoactive high of THC, it's considered a relatively safe drug. In fact, the World Health Organization (WHO) released a preliminary report in 2017 that stated, "CBD is generally well tolerated with a good safety profile."[376]

Many people claim they have also found benefits from CBN oil or blends of CBD and THC. Results vary and are dependent on a vast number of factors, including strain and the use of terpenes. Terpenes are aromatic oils that give each strain its own unique aroma, or flavor, and may provide enhanced medical benefits. As you can see, it's a complicated industry and just trying to understand the basics can create its own anxiety.

Still, a few things are essential to keep in mind. First, as I mentioned at the top, cannabis and its products are still illegal in many U.S. states and several other countries. If you wish to investigate cannabis as an option, please check your local laws to see if any of these products are legally available to you. Second, most people agree that the use of cannabis products during benzo use and/or taper is ill-advised. Some have found that the best effects are during the protracted stages of withdrawal, well after your last dose of benzos. Third, cannabis, like most psychoactive drugs, can be addictive, cause dependence, and have its own withdrawal complications.

Did you try any cannabis products for your withdrawal?

I happen to live in the majestic state of Colorado in the U.S. It just so happens that cannabis, both medical and recreational, is legal here. This allows me the luxury of trying this as an option.

Since my symptoms have carried on in a protracted state for a few years now, I decided to sample some cannabis compounds to see if they would help. I have tried a few different strains of CBD oil and even some blends with low-level THC. Unfortunately, the jury is still out on its effectiveness for me. I can't say that I've noticed any significant benefits or complications. I may keep experimenting, but part of me just wants to let my body finish its healing process on its own, unencumbered by any additional drugs.

But, before I move on, I do need to make this clear: As the author of this book, I do not endorse the use of cannabis products in any way, shape, or form. Especially if they're illegal in your area. Please be cautious if you wish to pursue this course of treatment.

What about other drugs?

Other medications might be contraindicated for those taking benzos, and you should consult with your doctor if you're concerned. They're too numerous for me to list here, but I do have a suggestion: Go through your medicine cabinet, including your vitamins and supplements, and list them out. Then, search *The Ashton Manual* and even the benzo boards for those medication names. Check if there are possible complications with them that someone else has noted. Then take that list into your next appointment with your doctor for discussion.

Just don't get too carried away. Remember that the anxiety created by worrying about all these complications can be worse than the complications themselves.

So, these are the boundaries. Did you discover any lasting benefits from the ones you set?

Quite a few, actually.

One of the best lessons I learned from my experience with benzo withdrawal is how to eat healthier. When your body is so overreactive to foods, you don't have much choice but to carefully analyze what you put into your body. I was never a salad eater. I would always choose a burger over veggies. Now, my most frequent dinner is a spinach salad that I make with almonds, blueberries, bell pepper, and anything else I can find in the crisper drawer. And the weird thing is, I like it. I enjoy a good salad and snacking on veggies. Trust me, I still eat a burger now and then, but far less than I used to. Reducing sugar, caffeine, and alcohol are other diet changes that I still embrace today.

What I'm trying to say here is that a few of the boundaries I set during withdrawal are healthy, long-term changes and have carried over into my life after I recovered. Some good came out of this crazy experience. It's something, and I'll take it.

Time to move on.

CHAPTER 15

THE NATURAL PATH

Are you going to get all holistic on me now?

Yes, but just stick with me for a bit. You might find it interesting.

Not likely, but I've come this far.

Thanks for the lackluster vote of confidence. I'll try and be quick.

It's only "natural" that many of us turn to alternative solutions to help with our condition during benzo withdrawal. Medical science, in the form of a little pill, is the cause of our pain and discomfort and it's difficult for us to trust the medical establishment again. As a result, many of us have turned to more natural or alternative options.

This was true in my case. I have always been somewhat open-minded in my approach to medicine and health. This made my interest in natural options a smoother transition than it might be for others. But even if you're not a fan of alternative therapies, you may have become anti-drug or even anti-doctor, as so many have during this time. If that is the case, then it may leave you few other options.

I'm going to talk about a few different tools, techniques, and ways of life that have helped me. I'm not saying they're the right choices for you. Only you can determine what is best for you and your recovery.

Let's start with one of my favorites: meditation.

I've heard of meditation, but it sounds a bit New-Agey for me.

Well, you're not alone in that feeling. I felt the same way. But meditation has been around a long, long time. Perhaps there's something to it.

You talk when you cease to be at peace with your thoughts. [377]

— Kahlil Gibran, *The Prophet*

If I had to pick one simple mental tool that meant the most to me throughout my withdrawal and in the years following, it would have to be meditation. I was never a mediator before benzo withdrawal. Sitting still was not something that appealed to me. I was always on the go and needed constant stimulation.

As I prepared for my taper, my doctor encouraged me to find ways of stabilizing my anxiety and fear. Around that time, more and more scientific studies were coming out about the benefits of meditation, so I thought I'd give it a try. I downloaded some guided meditations, found a few free podcasts, and even discovered some excellent resources at my local library. Their messages spoke to me and helped me ease into the practice. Each morning I would try to sit quietly, relax, and see if I could calm my mind.

Now, all that sounds good, but trust me when I say that this was not some overnight miracle. Meditation can be quite challenging, especially for some anxiety-prone, benzo-dependent, TV-addicted guy with ADHD. Not a great combination for sitting still and quieting my mind. But I didn't give up. For the past five years now, I have been meditating. And just like any skill, it continually takes practice.

It's easy to get down on yourself about your ability to meditate, but it's important to remember that meditation is more about the attempt than the result. In a standard meditation session of about 15–20 minutes, it's not uncommon for my mind to wander 20, 30, even 40 times. And that's okay.

I guess what I am trying to say here is that meditating is not easy.

It takes a lot of practice and diligence, and it may not be for everyone. But if you give it a chance — an honest chance — it just might help you get through the gauntlet of benzo withdrawal.

But I'm not a Buddhist.

So? Meditation can be as secular or as religious as you choose. Whether your meditation prays to a higher power or merely focuses on your breath, it can have the same benefits. It's a way to learn to focus and clear your mind. You can tailor that practice to fit your beliefs or keep it independent of your faith. That is up to you.

What type of meditation do you practice?

There are more "types" of meditation than you can imagine. Finding ones that work for you might take time. It did for me. There are all sorts of books, classes, and audio recordings on meditation that are easy to find. One of the latest additions to this list are meditation apps like *Headspace, Breathe,* and *Calm,* which have become hugely successful. I found breathing meditation, guided meditation, and loving-kindness (metta) meditation to be my favorites, which I can do while I'm sitting or walking.

But I don't have time to meditate.

Yes, you do.

Can you find five minutes each day? If you can't, then you really might want to look at your priorities and re-schedule a few things. While most experts say that 15, 20, or 30 minutes are ideal for a beginning meditation session, it may be hard for some people to make the time. So, let me share with you something that my therapist, Christine, taught me.

I was having trouble finding time to meditate. I wanted to meditate in the morning, but I was usually too overwhelmed with my to-do list for the day. It was a constant struggle to convince myself that I had time to sit quietly. So, Christine suggested that I try something different. She told me to try and meditate five minutes each day. If I chose to go longer, fine, but I just needed to commit to five minutes. I gave it a shot.

She was right. Even when I was swamped, I could still convince myself to take just five minutes so I could check it off my list. But the strange thing was, I rarely meditated only five minutes. Most times, I would sit there for 20 or 30 minutes and get in a full, deep meditation session. Motivating myself to sit and start was the hardest part.

I now love to meditate. And I look forward to it. Even my dog looks forward to it. When I'm ready for my meditation, I look at "Bear" — that's my dog — and say "wanna hang out with me?" I then head to the basement. Bear follows me down and lays next to me. In fact, if I forget one day, he reminds me. More than once, Bear has stood at the top of the basement stairs looking at me. Reminding me that it's time to meditate. How cool is that?

If you have never meditated before, but want to give it a chance, try this: Do a standard breathing meditation for just five minutes each day. Sit in a relaxed but upright position, clear your mind and focus on your breathing, and if your mind wanders off — which it will — notice it, without judgment, and gently bring your focus back to your breath. That's it. Do that five minutes each day for a week and see how you feel. Perhaps it will become a habit, as it did for me.

How does meditation differ from mindfulness?

A lot of people get mindfulness and meditation confused. Meditation is the actual practice of quieting the mind often through a sitting or walking practice. Mindfulness is learning to stay focused on the moment without judgment. It's about accepting the world around you and finding peace in that acceptance. It's not about thinking of the future, and it's not about living in the past. It's about living in the now. It's about being present. That's mindfulness.

Why would I want to focus on the now if I'm in the middle of benzo withdrawal? Shouldn't I focus on the future or the past, when things were or will be better?

That's a valid argument, but I found the opposite to be true.

Much of the emotional pain that I experienced during withdrawal was generated when I focused on the future or the past, not on the present. Mindfulness is not about running away from feelings, emotions, or even thoughts. It's about accepting everything as it is and not fighting against it. You might think that sounds counterintuitive with benzo withdrawal, but I would have to disagree.

So how do you be mindful?

You pay attention. You pay attention to what is happening right now in front of you.

I am king of not-being-in-the-moment. Trust me on this one. My brain doesn't help much either. I am almost always thinking of one thing, or three things, while doing another four things. But then again, aren't we all to some degree?

Mindfulness teaches us to focus on what we're doing right now, this very moment. Even if it's something trivial like eating, or walking, or brushing your teeth. Pay attention to what you're doing. Notice every little sensation. The color of the sky. The sound of the birds. The smell of the bread in the oven. The taste of an orange.

And as you notice that color, sound, smell, or taste, do it without judgment. Don't judge that color as good or bad; just see it. Don't judge that sound as sharp or flat; just hear it. We judge everything, and that judgment leads to suffering. The speed of communication in modern day life has only increased our insatiable desire to judge, and judge quickly. Recognizing this trait in yourself is an excellent first step in learning to lessen your own suffering.

Try to experience the world around you as it is. That is the essence of mindfulness.

You also mentioned yoga in the opening. Did you find that helpful in your recovery?

Yes. Definitely.

I'll first admit that I haven't been to a yoga class in a few months, and I'm not proud of it. But don't let that fool you. I'm a believer in yoga and would recommend it to anyone who asks. In fact, my wife and I are scheduled to start yoga back up this Friday, and I'm really looking forward to it.

I discovered yoga when I was stabilizing before starting my taper. I found a class at the local gym and loved it. It was a vinyasa type of yoga, and it was great for me. I also met and befriended a couple of people in the class who were struggling with benzos too. What a small world. After my wife and I moved into our new house, our local recreation center offered classes, and we became fans of Yin yoga, which is mostly deep stretching. In Yin, you hold each stretching position for three to five minutes. It's hard, but it works. This class has since been canceled, and I miss it.

There are all types of yoga classes for all types of needs. Hot yoga and core yoga are more geared towards cardio and fitness, while others like vinyasa and Yin are more focused on stretching and meditative practice. I got my cardio workout separately, so I usually preferred more meditative types of yoga, which helped my mind as well as my body. One of the most significant benefits of yoga for someone in withdrawal is the stretching. Our muscles are locked up and crave to be relaxed and loosened, and yoga is perfect for that. Tai Chi is a similar practice with much of the same benefits.

I won't go into too much detail on yoga here. If you're interested, check out a DVD at the library, visit YouTube, or take a class as I did. Remember, though, that during withdrawal our muscles can be very tight. As with exercise, make sure you ease into it and don't overdo it. Listen to your body and adjust. I think of yoga as therapy for both my mind and body. It's something kind I can do for myself during this trying time.

Did you ever try acupuncture?

Many recent studies have confirmed the benefits of acupuncture for anxiety and insomnia. I first tried acupuncture a few years ago while I was in acute withdrawal to help with my muscle tightness and pain. I had about six or seven sessions. I wasn't sure if it was helping me or not, and since I was starting up physical therapy, I decided to discontinue.

More recently, though, as I'm nearing completion of the book, I have decided to give acupuncture another chance. This time specifically for anxiety. I found a new acupuncturist, Kathryn, who specializes in Japanese Acupuncture. She has a very kind presence and puts me at ease during our sessions. I've only been to a few sessions so far, but I do think that it is helping. Perhaps my body is more responsive in protracted withdrawal than in acute. I'll continue for a while to see what the long-term benefits are. So far, I'm optimistic.

How about massage?

Massage has been a lasting favorite of mine. My massage therapist, Liz, is a semi-pro volleyball player and she can really work the deep tissues. She also became a friend and helped keep me motivated to write this book. Since I had constant muscle aches and pains throughout, her treatments became crucial to my recovery. I have an appointment next week, and I'm truly looking forward to it.

And what about spirituality? Did you find that helpful at all?

The last thing I want to do is proselytize in this book. I have a Protestant Christian background, and since I was an adult, I have been looking for a faith to call my own. I guess I would call myself a "seeker." While I do believe in God in some shape or form, I don't subscribe to any one dogma or religion. Therefore, I'm open to input from a lot of sources, and I'm very curious. I am also respectful of people's individual beliefs and their right to have them.

If you're a person of faith, then rely on that faith. It just might be the saving grace you're looking for during this trying time. And if you don't believe in a supreme being, then find support in your family, friends, or yourself. In the end, be true to you. That's what really matters. Find what works for you and stick with it.

Any other natural or non-drug treatments?

Absolutely. Aromatherapy, coloring books, dancing, drumming, essential oils, focused breathing, hydration, hygge, laughter, music, nature therapy, pet therapy, reading, singing, travel, touch, volunteering and about a hundred other ancient and modern techniques have been proven to help reduce anxiety and can aid your body in healing. I experimented with many of these at one point or another during my withdrawal and had some success. I wrote a whole chapter in detail on these techniques, but it got cut in the final draft. Perhaps it will resurface in my next book.

CHAPTER 16

FOR THE CAREGIVER

written by Shana Foster

What is this chapter about and who wrote it?

I had planned on writing a chapter for people who are caregivers to those of us going through benzo withdrawal. Unfortunately, I never got around to it, and during my final review, I felt it was suspiciously absent. And then, unprompted, my wife offered to write something for the book. I loved the idea and jumped on the opportunity. Who better to write this chapter than the person who had to put up with me going through withdrawal for five hard years.

This next section will diverge from the Q&A format temporarily to fit better with Shana's writing style. I'll pick it up again in the closing chapter that follows.

— D

Introduction

Benzodiazepine withdrawal syndrome (BWS) affects more than just the patients suffering from it. Although not in the same way or to the same extent, family members and friends — I'll call caregivers — are impacted by it as well. As a caregiver, you may find yourself unexpectedly comforting your loved one, dealing with personality changes, talking through symptoms and ways to mitigate them, altering routines, and canceling plans. Along the way, you and the person going through BWS may feel the effects of isolation, loss of normalcy, and perhaps lack of income if he or she is unable to work.

As D's wife, I can tell you that patience, understanding, reassurance, and flexibility are all keys to helping someone go through the difficult journey of recovery. Although I can't speak with any clinical expertise, I have learned some valuable lessons along the way that may be of help to those suffering from withdrawal symptoms and their friends and family members watching from the sidelines.

Believe the symptoms are real.

As D mentioned, most physical, emotional, and psychological symptoms of benzo withdrawal are invisible to others. For those of us on the outside, it's easy to doubt whether the symptoms are real, imagined, or invented to solicit sympathy or get out of doing an unpleasant activity. This can be terribly frustrating to those suffering from it. It's bad enough to go through benzo withdrawal, but then for others to question its existence makes it much worse. The single best thing you can do for those going through BWS is to provide assurance that you believe them.

Create a calm environment.

Since benzos are an anti-anxiety medication, it makes sense that people may experience more anxiety as they withdraw from the drug. At the same time, they might often be managing a myriad of physical symptoms, which only adds to their anxiety. That's even more reason they need to surround themselves with calming influences. And you can help with that.

Start with the obvious, like creating a quiet haven that can be mostly free of interruptions. Allow this to be a special place where the patient can escape for a while. Declutter your home so there are fewer obstacles that can cause frustration. Turn on relaxing music. Watch light-hearted movies. Go for nature walks. Listen more. Talk less.

Lighten the schedule. Plan ahead to avoid last-minute rushes.

Just don't make the place so comfy that he or she won't want to come out of it. When the symptoms subside, you may want to balance the isolation with some social experiences. I'll cover that shortly.

Allow for plenty of time and space.

Meditation and an afternoon nap have done wonders for my husband. He needs time to quiet his mind and body. Exercise has helped him manage his akathisia symptoms. He has been great about taking time for himself to do these things. But, sometimes life gets in the way, and it's easy to miss a session or two. When he starts to get easily agitated, I encourage him to take a few minutes for himself no matter the setting. This may mean that he escapes to the bedroom for 15 minutes while my family is visiting. Or, he stays in the car after we arrive at an event and joins me 10 minutes later. If he's feeling restless, taking a walk, exercising on the elliptical, or playing the drums have helped him.

Carefully time bringing up topics that trigger anxiety.

In keeping with a calm environment, as much as possible, try to avoid topics and situations that increase your loved one's anxiety when he or she is already in an agitated state. Wait until the symptoms subside so he or she can focus on the bigger picture.

For example, when D is restless and struggling with anxiety, that's not the time to talk about the in-laws coming to stay for a week or our need to save more for retirement. I wait a few hours — or perhaps the next day — until his symptoms diminish before broaching the subject.

Get back to the basics. Simplify.

Life is full of choices, distractions, and variables. For someone with BWS, it can be overwhelming and trigger anxiety. When that happens, I have found that it helps to limit the choices to two simpler options: Instead of, "We could go to the ballgame, plant a garden, watch a movie, have lunch at our favorite restaurant, host a BBQ with our friends, or go to the zoo with our cousins" I narrow it down to, "Would you rather go out or stay home?"

Here's an example of how that's played out for us. We were planning a trip to visit D's family, which is a 10-hour drive away. We've taken the route dozens of times before and always in one day. But when benzo anxiety and symptoms kicked in, the drive suddenly felt overwhelming to my husband. Rather than push the issue and create even more anxiousness, I suggested that we stop at a hotel part-way. As soon as I did, I saw his symptoms dramatically improve over a period of 60 seconds. Could we have driven it in one day? Certainly. But, I had a much calmer husband along the route, and that was worth it.

Prepare for potential personality changes, both good and bad.

For the first several years of my marriage to D, he was an easy-going guy. Sure, there were a couple of topics that would irritate him, but generally, he went with the flow. Then came benzos.

During the time he took clonazepam, I observed him becoming more anxious with each passing year. The anxiety exacerbated his ADHD symptoms, and he seemed to thrive on chaos, all the while getting more and more stressed. At its worst, I recall an example in the fall of 2010.

D is a big NFL football fan and was the commissioner for a fantasy league. On Sundays, he would set up camp in front of our 46-inch flat-screen TV. On the armrest of the chair, he would balance his laptop while his iPad rested in his lap. All three screens were set to different football games so he could keep track of his score in real-time. He was so stressed out as he tried to follow each player and game, but because it was football, he thought he was having fun.

Meanwhile, he was short-tempered with me, the dog, the doorbell, and anything else that dared interrupt him. His folks happened to be visiting at that time, and they noticed it too. In fact, my father-in-law pulled me aside and expressed sincere concern.

To be honest, this was just one example of how he was behaving all the time. My once easy-going husband had become an irritable guy who interrupted others, always seemed to be in a hurry, and tried to control each situation — including how I drove the car. It was clear that any comments or questions I had for him better be quick and to the point. And my car route must be direct and efficient.

The good news is that after D was off benzos for about a year, I began to see glimpses of the old easy-going guy again. It certainly helped that he was studying mindfulness and doing yoga. Over time, he has become more mild-tempered than he has been in a long time. He listens better. He doesn't try to hurry me through a story anymore. He isn't as critical of me. While he is more anxious at times and still struggles with protracted withdrawal, it's been a good change.

As your loved one goes through the waves and windows of benzo withdrawal, you may witness personality changes as well.

Budget for potential financial changes.

Some people go through BWS without missing work. For others, the symptoms are too intense to concentrate, and they need to step away from their jobs for a while. BWS symptoms are seemingly unpredictable and non-linear — symptoms don't necessarily clear up and go away entirely, like when you recover from the common cold. They seem to appear, disappear, and come back again later — a pattern known as waves and windows. So, even if your loved one is managing his or her symptoms effectively today, that doesn't necessarily mean that he or she won't need to miss work when the next wave of symptoms comes around. Either way, it's good to be prepared.

If the patient can't work, the loss of a regular income can have a big impact on finances. It might help to reduce unnecessary costs and save money during the smoother sailing times in case rough waters lie ahead. If there's any financial upside to BWS, it might be that your loved one spends less than usual because he or she doesn't feel up to going out as often. Then again, more frequent doctor visits might cancel that gain.

Let your friends and family members know what's happening.

Unfortunately, BWS is still relatively unknown to the general public. And since it's virtually invisible to others and can last for so long, it's easy to misunderstand the person going through it, doubt the condition is real, or even forget his symptoms exist. Heck, D and I spend nearly 24 hours per day under the same roof since we both work from home, and I still forget that he's struggling!

So, it's good to let your trusted friends and family members know what's happening and remind them of it periodically. This isn't like strep throat that goes away after a couple of weeks. When your friends and family are in the know, they tend to be much more understanding when you can't attend an event or cancel or change plans at the last minute. It's important for them to know that sometimes the physical or emotional symptoms of benzo withdrawal make it difficult or impossible for the patient to leave the house and/or be around other people.

Be flexible and invent alternatives.

Since BWS symptoms are unpredictable, it's not uncommon for them to flare up at the worst possible times. Perhaps you've made long-awaited plans to see *Hamilton* when it comes to town, but your loved one just doesn't feel up to it. Sure, it's disappointing, but you can make the best of it.

If the plans can't be changed, go anyway and allow him or her to rest at home. Or, reschedule for another time. If the patient is up to it, suggest a new activity that will work for everyone involved. For example, my husband and I had plans to go on a hike with a friend, but the thought of walking along a rocky path with his groin pain and benzo belly was more than he could handle. So, we suggested instead that the friend join us for pizza and games at our home so my husband could be more relaxed in a comfortable setting while still socializing together.

Another example is when we had tickets for a winter sleigh ride in Breckenridge, Colorado, with a group of our neighbors. We had hotel reservations and planned to make a weekend of it. My husband's symptoms — and his anxiety about potential symptoms — kept increasing as the time grew nearer. So, I invited my niece to go in his place. My husband was relieved, and it gave me an opportunity to get to know my niece better.

Remember, it's the condition and not the person.

Okay, so between us, there are certainly times when my patience grows thin. Like when I've developed cabin fever because my husband hasn't felt up to going out for the past three weeks. Or, he's frustrated with me because he feels blindsided when his benzo-fogged brain doesn't recall an important detail even though I shared it with him twice before. Or, he wants to talk through his symptoms and possible causes for the gazillionth time. Or, he doesn't feel good, and it seems like he's taking it out on me. Or, I wonder if maybe he's exaggerating his symptoms to get out of going to an event he doesn't really want to attend anyway. I've been there. At times like these, it's more difficult to feel the loving compassion for him. When I hit a wall, I get away for a while to blow off some steam.

What helps me in moments like these is to remember the guy behind the symptoms. This isn't him — it's his condition that's causing him to be more emphatic, anxious, forgetful, irritated, or withdrawn. When I think of it that way, it helps me find the compassion I need and rekindles the love I have for him. This journey isn't easy for me. It's even harder for him.

Focus on what the patient can do.

It's understandable that people going through BWS may get down on themselves because of their limitations. Perhaps their diet is super restrictive, which has a huge impact on attending social events. Or, maybe going to the planetarium isn't an option because they can't sit still for that long because their body won't stop twitching. Benzo withdrawal offers plenty of opportunities to say no and dwell on what you can't do. Instead, help your loved one focus on what he or she can do.

Is it difficult to attend a church potluck because of food sensitivities? That's okay, just eat before you go and mingle around the party with a glass of water in your hand. Nobody will notice anyway. Or, is attending your son's entire baseball game too overwhelming? No problem, walk the fence line while you watch him play, disappear for a bit during the third inning to meditate, or attend what you can and come back later. Is working outside the home too much to handle?

Find things to do around the house that bring a sense of purpose and accomplishment. Start small if you must, like taking out the trash, fixing the broken lamp, or raking the yard.

Find gratitude.

When I'm suffering, it's easy to think that I have it worse than anyone else in the history of the world. But that's not true. It helps to remember that some others have much greater challenges and manage to not only get through the day but in some cases thrive. Think Michael J. Fox with his Parkinson's disease, or the military veteran who lost both legs in Iraq and now inspires others with his story.

Despite the circumstances, somebody always has it worse than the person going through BWS. Together with your loved one, you can be grateful that you both can feed yourselves, walk through the grocery store, smell and taste the warm bread, and see the fresh buds on the crabapple tree outside the window. Practice looking for the positive each day. There's so much to be grateful for, but it's easy to put on blinders when you're in pain. When you and the patient think of the positive aspects of your lives, it helps you both feel better despite your circumstances.

Take care of yourself.

As a caregiver, it's easy to get sucked into the overwhelming vortex of symptoms, anxiety, and sense of helplessness that accompanies benzo withdrawal. It's important to keep yourself in a healthy state of mind. After all, how effective can you be as a caregiver if you're frazzled, depressed, and bitter?

Here are three things that have helped me maintain or regain some sanity:

Balance comfort with "me time." BWS can be overwhelming for the person going through it. When symptoms are at their worst, it's easy to devote your entire day to comforting the patient. But, work, laundry, dishes, taking your daughter to a birthday party, picking up your son from practice, etc. still must be done. And, you need to take time for yourself amid it all. Sometimes, your loved one might appreciate your presence 24/7, while other times he or she might prefer to be alone. Either way, it's good to give the patient time and space to work through symptoms on his or her own. Find a balance that works for both of you.

Go for a change of scenery. Cabin fever can set up quickly when you and your loved one spend all your time at home. It's understandable — when you don't feel good, there's no place better than home. But after a while, it's healthy to experience new sites, smells, and sounds. Start small, like a trip to the grocery store or walk around the neighborhood. On better days, try strolling around the mall or going out to eat. It's amazing how getting away from the routine can help lift both of your spirits.

Avoid isolation. It's understandable that benzo withdrawal symptoms can force the biggest of extroverts into hiding. Will they feel up to socializing? What if their symptoms kick in during dinner? Will the friends or family understand? Won't it be embarrassing to have to leave the show half-way into the second act? These fears are quite real and make it so tempting to stay home alone. But, it's good to interact with others and maintain relationships. And, if for no other reason, it's good for them to think about something else besides their own symptoms for a while. Encourage your loved one to socialize with friends and family as much as his or her symptoms will allow. If it's better to stay home, invite the friends to come over. If the patient needs to excuse him or herself for a few minutes to lay down, your friends will understand.

Your need for socialization is important too. It's tempting to stay home with the patient instead of venturing out with friends and family members throughout the withdrawal process. After several months, you might find that your own relationships with others feel more distant. It's important to maintain your own support system for times when you need a shoulder to cry on, distraction, or advice.

Summary

Benzo withdrawal can turn peoples' lives up-side-down, which can have a direct impact on those around them — including you. By believing them, creating a calm environment, simplifying, focusing on the positive, and taking time for yourself, you and your loved one can weather the storms more comfortably.

CHAPTER 17

BENZO FREE

As you look back at your withdrawal, do you feel there are benefits to this experience?

There are benefits to everything in life. Learning is often one of the most significant gains. In fact, we usually learn the most from the negative events in our life, not from the positive. We would never grow if all of life's experiences were pleasant. Benzo withdrawal is a journey just like life, and as with all adventures, it has its highs and its lows.

The truth is, benzo withdrawal lowered the bar for my expectations in life. Sounds kind of depressing, doesn't it? It's funny, but I don't see it that way. It's all about perspective. I still have dreams of what I want to accomplish and experience, but at the same time, I get more enjoyment out of the little things now. An evening reading in front of the fire with my wife and dog. A long walk at twilight. Watching my nephew's baseball game or listening to my niece play the piano. Writing this book. Sure, there's a lot more out there in life, and perhaps I'll get to experience some of it in the coming years. But I've been to hell and back through benzo withdrawal, and that perspective has made my life right now look damn good.

And that perspective shift wasn't the only benefit. I lost weight and became a much healthier eater. I now exercise more and enjoy a more active lifestyle. I don't worry as much about the little aches and pains along the way. I cherish my family and friends more and make sure that I let them know that. I now dream and can enjoy the luxury of an occasional seven-hour night's sleep. I now feel. That's a big one. I feel.

Are you referring to returning emotions?

Exactly. This is one of those benefits.

As I mentioned earlier, when you go through withdrawal, and the drugs that have been numbing your nervous system ease their control, something bizarre starts to happen. Emotions come back. Sometimes with a vengeance. And for me, with all those emotions, came the irrepressible desire to cry. Sounds crazy for a 52-year-old man to say that, doesn't it? Well, perhaps that is part of the problem.

> *Heaven knows we need never be ashamed of our tears, for they are rain upon the blinding dust of earth, overlying our hard hearts. I was better after I had cried, than before — more sorry, more aware of my own ingratitude, more gentle.* [378]

— Charles Dickens, *Great Expectations*

Most of us were taught not to cry as children. Men probably more than women, but I know a few women who also struggle with this issue. It doesn't really matter the gender. All that matters is that somehow we got the message that crying was not acceptable. And that real men, or real women, don't cry. Whether it was from our parents, peers, society, or the media; it was hard not to get the message.

And I get it. You can't have a soldier break down and cry on the front lines of the battlefield if you expect to win the war. In fact, even in the workplace, we wouldn't get a lot done if everyone started crying at every little incident of displeasure or criticism. That is not the crying I am talking about. I'm speaking about the deep emotions that have been internalized over years and years of suppression. The dam we built holding back decades of pain and tears.

About 12 years ago, my father was diagnosed with prostate cancer. It was stage three and, although he had excellent treatment, there was a chance that he wouldn't make it. Thank God, we were blessed, and my father is still with us to this day. But what I carry away from that experience more than anything else is the positive change that my dad experienced. My dad, the strong, masculine man that I looked up to — and still do to this day — started to cry. The dam burst, and the tears began to fall. Decades of repressed sadness and frustration came flooding out. All the pain and stress and hurt and loss. All that emotion had been bottled up inside, and it finally came out.

And you know what? It was one of the greatest things that ever happened to him. Over time, the crying subsided, but he still cries now and then. And I'm glad. I encourage it and tell him it's okay every time he does. He needs it.

So, when I went through benzo withdrawal, I was prepared. Or I thought I was. I, too, lived most of my life unable to cry. But when I started withdrawal, the floodgates opened for me, just as they did for my dad. I can't tell you the number of times I sobbed on my wife's shoulder. Hell, I just broke down two days ago with a good cry. Some of it was about the benzos, but most of it was crap that had been stuffed deep inside from decades ago.

I now love to cry. I do. Being sad is not an inherently bad thing. Feeling the sadness is healthy. Letting the emotion out is healthy. If I don't want to die of a heart attack at 55, I must learn to let the stress find its release. In fact, if I feel the emotion start to build over a week or so, I'll even watch a sad movie just to instigate the release. And the best part is that after that cry, I feel better. Unfortunately, the dam that took decades to build doesn't get destroyed all at once. I can't just cry at will. It's still hard to do. But slowly, ever so slowly, I'm tearing down that dam. I still might hide in my closet so nobody sees me, but I do cry, and I'm okay with that.

Allow the feelings to come. Accept them, don't fight them. I try not to ruminate on them too much, but I allow them to come, and I allow them to pass. We are human, and we feel. And as we remove the drugs that suppressed these emotions from our systems, our feelings are free to flow again. And that is a good thing.

What other benefits did you have?

As I've noted several times in this book, I read and researched extensively during withdrawal. I learned about benzos, about mindfulness and meditation, about happiness, about health and medicine, and so much more. This learning is a huge gain for me. It has not only helped me write this book but has also prepared me for helping others who are struggling with the same experience.

I also learned about my relationships. While withdrawal is an excellent tool for determining the strength and durability of our own resolve, the same can be said of our bonds with others. Going through difficult times, such as benzo withdrawal, can bring some people in our lives closer to us while driving others away. It provides a looking glass through which we can see past the facade of superficial connections and peak at the underlying infrastructure and stability of our relationships.

Withdrawal can be almost as demanding on the caretaker or loved one as it is on the patient. Finding someone who will stick it out with us is an incredible ask. I can't imagine what this experience over the past five-plus years has been like for my wife. Supporting me medically, emotionally, and financially has been a considerable burden and she has carried it like a champ. I know it was not easy. Far from it. I hate that my dependence has done this to her and I am hopeful it will end soon.

One change that neither of us expected was the change in my personality as Shana mentioned in chapter 16. Benzo withdrawal can be a significant life event, and people who face events like this often find subtle, and even not-so-subtle, differences in their personality. I am a different person now. Maybe not significantly, but noticeably. My wife and family see the changes more than I do, and they agree that most of them are for the better. While I'm not a fan of the increased anxiety, irritability, and some other lingering symptoms, I am quite fond of being a better husband. Shana tells me I'm quieter now. More thoughtful and introspective. I listen better to her and to others. Benzo withdrawal has brought us closer together, and I'll be eternally grateful for that gift.

Trust me, I'm not volunteering to do this withdrawal thing over again. But I do see the forest for the trees. I am a better person because of my withdrawal from benzodiazepines. It forced me to take a long hard look at my life and find a better way to live. I am grateful for that. And that's the truth.

Any last encouraging words?

It's sad to think that our conversation has reached its conclusion, but all things must come to an end.

I never once regretted my decision to withdraw from benzos. Even though I am in protracted withdrawal, still have symptoms, still struggle with anxiety and cognitive function, and still have bad days; it was the best choice I ever made. But that is me. This is about you, and the decision is yours. Don't let anyone force you to withdraw until you are ready. But, if you choose to withdraw, once you're benzo-free, know this:

Life is better on the other side.
Much better.

I am no longer controlled by some medication. I may not have my old life back, but I don't really want it anymore. I have a new life. And a new me. My marriage survived the ordeal even better than before. I learned so much, and I am so much stronger than I ever was. I'm here, and I've found the joy of being benzo-free.

Prof. Ashton reminds us that anyone can withdraw from benzos who really wants to, and I totally agree. You can do this. All of us who have gone before you believe in you and are here to guide you along the way.

Relax, let yourself heal, and taper slowly,
D

APPENDIX

Types of Benzos

The following list includes most benzodiazepines, z-drugs, and thienodiazepines on the market today and lists their generic name followed by most common brand name and other information, if available. *The Ashton Manual* is the primary source for this data, supplemented by The National Health Service (NHS), the NIH's Pub Chem Open Chemistry Database, and others.[379] Values for half-life and other data points can vary significantly based on source and by individual.

LEGEND

Onset – The duration of time until the drug initially takes effect.

Half-Life – The amount of time it takes for half of the initial dose to be left in the blood. Active metabolite is shown in square brackets if available.

Equivalency (potency) – The equivalency value is as compared to 10 mg of diazepam. For example, 0.5 mg of alprazolam roughly equals 10 mg of diazepam. Thus, the lower the equivalency value, the higher the potency of the drug.

This is not a complete list of benzos and is provided for informational purposes only. **It should not be used as a basis for substitution calculations or for any other medical use.** *Any reduction in dosage should only be made under direct supervision of a licensed physician.*

Benzodiazepines

Adinazolam (Deracyn)
Market Focus: Anxiety / Depression
Onset: Intermediate
Half-life: 3 hours

Alprazolam (Xanax)
Other Brand Names: Alprax,, Alprox, Alprocontin, Alzam, Alzolam, Anzilum, Apo-Alpraz, Helex, Kalma, Misar, Mylan-Alprazolam, Neurol, Niravam, Novo-Alprazol, Nu-Alpraz, Onax, Pacyl, Restyl, Solanax, Tafil, Tranax, Trankimazin, Trika, Xycalm, Xanor, Zolam, Zopax
Market Focus: Anxiety / Depression
Onset: Intermediate
Half-life: 6–12 hours
Equivalency: 0.5 mg

Bromazepam (Lexotan)
Other Brand Names: Brazepam, Bromam, Bromaze, Lectopam, Lexatin, Lexaurin, Lexilium, Lexomil, Lexotanil, Rekotnil, Somalium
Market Focus: Anxiety / Insomnia / Amnesia (Surgical)
Onset: Intermediate
Half-life: 10–20 hours
Equivalency: 5-6 mg

Camazepam (Paxor)
Other Brand Names: Albego, Limpidon
Market Focus: Anxiety
Onset: Short
Half-life: 6–30 hours

Chlordiazepoxide (Librium)
Other Brand Names: Apo-chlordiazepoxide, Corax, Elenium, Medilium, Nova-Pam, Nova-Poxide, Risolid, Solium
Market Focus: Anxiety / Alcohol Withdrawal
Onset: Long
Half-life: 5–30 hours [36–200 hours]
Equivalency: 25 mg

Cinolazepam (Gerodorm)
Market Focus: Insomnia
Onset: Short
Half-life: 9 hours

Clobazam (Frisium)
Other Brand Names: Onfi, Tapclob, Urbanol
Market Focus: Anxiety / Seizures
Onset: Intermediate
Half-life: 12–60 hours
Equivalency: 20 mg

Clonazepam (Klonopin)
Other Brand Names: Iktorivil, Paxam, Rivatril, Rivotril
Market Focus: Anxiety / Seizures / Muscle Relaxant
Onset: Intermediate
Half-life: 18–50 hours
Equivalency: 0.5 mg

Clorazepate (Tranxene)
Other Brand Names: Apo-Clorazepate, Gen-Xene, Novo-Clopate, Tranxillium
Market Focus: Anxiety / Seizures
Onset: Long
Half-life: [36–200 hours]
Equivalency: 15 mg

Cloxazolam (Akton)
Other Brand Names: Lubalix, Olcadil, Sepazon
Market Focus: Anxiety / Seizures
Onset: Long
Half-life: 65 hours

Delorazepam (Dadumir)
Other Brand Names: EN
Market Focus: Anxiety / Amnesia (Surgical)
Onset: Intermediate
Half-life: 80–115 hours

Diazepam (Valium)
Other Brand Names: Antenex, Apaurin, Apo-Diazepam, Apozepam, Apzepam, D-Pam, Diazemuls, Diazepan, Ducene, E Pam, Hexalid, Meval, Normabel, Novo-Diapam, Pax, PMS-Diazepam, Pro-Pam, Stesolid, Vival, Vivol, Valaxona
Market Focus: Anxiety / Seizures / Muscle Relaxant
Onset: Long
Half-life: 20–100 hours [36-200 hours]
Equivalency: 10 mg

Estazolam (ProSam)
Other Brand Names: Nuctalon, Tasedan
Market Focus: Anxiety / Insomnia
Onset: Intermediate
Half-life: 10–24 hours
Equivalency: 1-2 mg

Ethyl Loflazepate (Victan)
Other Brand Names: Meliax, Ronlax
Market Focus: Anxiety
Onset: Long
Half-life: 70–120 hours

Flunitrazepam (Rohypnol)
Other Brand Names: Flunipam, Fluscand, Hipnosedon, Hypnodorm, Rohydorm, Rohypnol, Ronal, Vulbegal
Market Focus: Insomnia
Onset: Short
Half-life: 18–26 hours [36–200 hours]
Equivalency: 1 mg

Flurazepam (Dalmane)
Other Brand Names: Apo-Flurazepam, Dalmadorm, Fluzepam, Novo-Flupam, PMS-Flupam, Som Pam, Somnol
Market Focus: Insomnia
Onset: Long
Half-life: [40–250 hours]
Equivalency: 15-30 mg

Flutazolam (Coreminal)
Market Focus: Insomnia
Onset: Short
Half-life: 4 hours

Flutoprazepam (Restas)
Market Focus: Insomnia / Seizures
Onset: Intermediate
Half-life: 60–90 hours

Halazepam (Paxipam)
Market Focus: Anxiety
Onset: Intermediate
Half-life: [30–100 hours]
Equivalency: 20 mg

Haloxazolam (Somelin)
Market Focus: Anxiety

Ketazolam (Anxon)
Other Brand Names: Solatran
Market Focus: Anxiety
Onset: Long
Half-life: 30–100 hours [36–200 hours]
Equivalency: 15-30 mg

Loprazolam (Dormonoct)
Market Focus: Insomnia
Onset: Short
Half-life: 6–12 hours
Equivalency: 1-2 mg

Lorazepam (Ativan)
Other Brand Names: Apo-Lorazepam, Lorabenz, Lorenin, Lorsilan, Novo-Lorazepam, Nu-Loraz, Orfidal, PMS-Lorazepam, Pro-Lorazepam, Tavor, Temesta
Market Focus: Anxiety / Insomnia / Seizures / Muscle Relaxant / Amnesia (Surgical)
Onset: Intermediate
Half-life: 10–20 hours
Equivalency: 1 mg

Lormetazepam (Noctamid)
Other Brand Names: Loramet, Pronoctan
Market Focus: Insomnia
Onset: Intermediate
Half-life: 10–12 hours
Equivalency: 1-2 mg

Medazepam (Nobrium)
Other Brand Names: Ansilan, Mezapam, Raporan, Rudotel
Market Focus: Anxiety
Onset: Intermediate
Half-life: 30–200 hours
Equivalency: 10 mg

Mexazolam (Sedexil)
Other Brand Names: Melex
Market Focus: Anxiety
Onset: Intermediate

Midazolam (Versed)
Other Brand Names: Dormicum, Dormonid, Hypnovel
Market Focus: Insomnia / Seizures / Amnesia (Surgical)
Onset: Short
Half-life: 1–6 hours
Equivalency: 7 mg (oral)

Nimetazepam (Erimin)
Market Focus: Insomnia
Onset: Short
Half-life: 14–30 hours

Nitrazepam (Mogadon)
Other Brand Names: Alodorm, Dumolid, Insomna, Nitrados, Nitrazadon, Pacisyn
Market Focus: Insomnia / Seizures
Onset: Intermediate
Half-life: 15–38 hours
Equivalency: 10 mg

Nordazepam / Nordiazepam (Nordaz)
Other Brand Names: Calmday, Madar, Stilny
Market Focus: Anxiety
Onset: Long
Half-life: 30–200 hours
Equivalency: 10 mg

Oxazepam (Serax)
Other Brand Names: Alepam, Apo-Oxazepam, Benzotran, Murelax, Novo-Oxazepam, Opamox, Oxabenz, Oxapax, Oxascand, Oxpam, PMS-Oxazepam, Serafax, Serapax, Serenid, Seresta, Sobril, Zapex
Market Focus: Anxiety
Onset: Intermediate
Half-life: 4–15 hours
Equivalency: 20 mg

Phenazepam (Phenazepam)
Market Focus: Anxiety
Onset: Long
Half-life: 60 hours

Pinazepam (Domar)
Other Brand Names: Duna
Market Focus: Anxiety
Onset: Long
Half-life: 40–100 hours

Prazepam (Centrax)
Other Brand Names: Lysanxia
Market Focus: Anxiety
Onset: Long
Half-life: [36–200 hours]
Equivalency: 10-20 mg

Quazepam (Doral)
Market Focus: Insomnia
Onset: Intermediate
Half-life: 25–100 hours
Equivalency: 20 mg

Temazepam (Restoril)
Other Brand Names: Euhypnos, Nocturne, Normison, Sompam, Temaze, Temtabs, Tenox
Market Focus: Anxiety / Insomnia / Muscle Relaxant
Onset: Intermediate
Half-life: 8–22 hours
Equivalency: 20 mg

Tetrazepam (Myolastan)
Market Focus: Muscle Relaxant
Onset: Intermediate
Half-life: 3–24 hours

Triazolam (Halcion)
Other Brand Names: Apo-Triazo, Gen-Triazolam, Hypam, Novo-Triolam, Rilamir, Tricam
Market Focus: Insomnia
Onset: Short
Half-life: 2 hours
Equivalency: 0.5 mg

Nonbenzodiazepines (z-drugs)

Eszopiclone (Lunesta)
Market Focus: Insomnia
Onset: Short
Half-life: 6 hours (9 in elderly)
Equivalency: 3 mg

Zaleplon (Sonata)
Other Brand Names: Stamoc
Market Focus: Insomnia
Onset: Short
Half-life: 2 hours
Equivalency: 20 mg

Zolpidem (Ambien)
Other Brand Names: Nytamel, Sanval, Stilnoct, Stilnox, Sublinox, Xolnox, Zoldem, Zolnod
Market Focus: Insomnia
Onset: Short
Half-life: 2 hours
Equivalency: 20 mg

Zopiclone (Zimovane)
Other Brand Names: Imovane, Rhovane, Ximovan, Zileze, Zimoclone, Zopiklone, Zopitan, Zorclone
Market Focus: Insomnia
Onset: Short
Half-life: 5–6 hours
Equivalency: 15 mg

Thienodiazepines

Bentazepam (Thiadipona)
Market Focus: Anxiety
Onset: Intermediate
Half-life: 2–4 hours

Brotizolam (Lendormin)
Other Brand Names: Dormex, Sintonal, Noctilan
Market Focus: Insomnia
Onset: Short
Half-life: 4–5 hours

Clotiazepam (Clozan)
Other Brand Names: Rize, Veratran
Market Focus: Anxiety
Onset: Intermediate
Half-life: 4 hours

Etizolam (Depax)
Other Brand Names: Etilaam, Etizest, ETizola, Pasaden
Market Focus: Anxiety / Insomnia / Seizures / Muscle Relaxant / Amnesia (Surgical)
Onset: Intermediate
Half-life: 6 hours

Resources

The following resources are listed as a courtesy and are for informational purposes only. They do not constitute an endorsement or approval by the author or publisher for any information, products, advice, or services contained therein.

THE ASHTON MANUAL

Benzodiazepines: How They Work and How to Withdraw (aka The Ashton Manual)
www.benzo.org.uk/manual
THE resource guide for benzodiazepine withdrawal.

SUICIDE PREVENTION

United States

Emergency Services (U.S. & Canada)
911

National Suicide Prevention Lifeline
Call 800-273-TALK(8255)
www.suicidepreventionlifeline.org
The National Suicide Prevention Lifeline is a national network of local crisis centers that provides free and confidential emotional support to people in suicidal crisis or emotional distress 24 hours a day, 7 days a week.

Crisis Text Line
Text HOME to 741741
www.crisistextline.org
Crisis Text Line is free, 24/7 support for those in crisis. Text 741741 from anywhere in the U.S. to text with a trained crisis counselor.

The Trevor Project
Call 866-488-7386 or Text "Trevor" to 202-304-1200
www.thetrevorproject.org
The Trevor Project is the leading national organization providing crisis intervention and suicide prevention services to lesbian, gay, bisexual, transgender, and questioning (LGBTQ) young people ages 13–24.

Veterans Crisis Line
Call 800-273-8255 (Press 1) or Text 838255
www.veteranscrisisline.net
The Veterans Crisis Line connects veterans in crisis and their families and friends with qualified, caring Department of Veterans Affairs responders through a confidential toll-free hotline, online chat, or text.

United Kingdom

Emergency Services (U.K.)
999 / 111

Samaritans
Call 116 123 (UK & ROI)
www.samaritans.org
A 24/7 crisis line for immediate support. Founded in 1953, Samaritans has 201 branches across the U.K. and Republic of Ireland.

Papyrus: Prevention of Young Suicide
Call 0800 068 4141
www.papyrus-uk.org
Papyrus draws from the experience of many who have been touched personally by young suicide across the U.K. and speaks on their behalf.

Campaign Against Living Miserably (CALM)
Call 0800 58 58 58 (nationwide) or 0808 802 58 58 (London)
www.thecalmzone.net
This helpline is for men in the U.K. who are down or have hit a wall for any reason, who need to talk or find information and support. They're open 5pm–midnight, 365 days a year.

Mind
Call 0300 123 3393 or Text 86463
www.mind.org.uk
Mind provides advice and support to empower anyone experiencing a mental health problem. They campaign to improve services, raise awareness and promote understanding. Lines are open 9am to 6pm, Monday to Friday (except for bank holidays).

Other Countries

International Association for Suicide Prevention (IASP)

www.iasp.info/resources/Crisis_Centres
This resource provides a clickable map to find worldwide crisis centers.

Wikipedia List of Worldwide Suicide Crisis Lines

en.wikipedia.org/wiki/List_of_suicide_crisis_lines
Wikipedia provides a list of suicide crisis lines from several countries around the world.

BENZODIAZEPINE SUPPORT GROUPS

Benzo Withdrawal Information

Battle Against Tranquillisers (BAT)

www.bataid.org
BAT helps those who are addicted to benzodiazepines, z-drug tranquillisers, and sleeping pills (and drugs with similar effects) and who wish to withdraw from them.

Benzo Free

www.benzofree.org
The *Benzo Free* website is dedicated to those who suffer from benzodiazepine dependence. Services include the "Benzo Free Podcast," a resource link database, and a variety of other services. This site is also the official website for this book.

benzo.org.uk

www.benzo.org.uk
Home to *The Ashton Manual*, benzo.org.uk is dedicated to sufferers of iatrogenic benzodiazepine tranquilliser addiction. Launched on July 6, 2000, this website has always been a work in progress, consisting of articles, information, expert medical documents, news stories, and personal accounts.

BenzoBuddies

www.benzobuddies.org
An inclusive, nonjudgmental mutual-support environment for those who wish to withdraw from benzodiazepines. Members of the BenzoBuddies community are encouraged to exchange ideas, information, and support during the process of withdrawal and recovery.

Benzodiazepine Information Coalition (BIC)

www.benzoinfo.com

Benzodiazepine Information Coalition is a non-profit organization that advocates for a greater understanding of the potentially devastating effects of commonly prescribed benzodiazepines.

Bristol & District Tranquilliser Project (BTP)
www.btpinfo.org.uk
Originally founded in 1985 as a tranquilliser withdrawal group, the Bristol & District Tranquilliser Project is a voluntary organization set up to help people who are experiencing involuntary addiction to prescribed minor tranquillisers, sleeping pills, and antidepressants.

World Benzodiazepine Awareness Day (W-BAD)
www.w-bad.org
World Benzodiazepine Awareness Day seeks to raise global awareness about the severe problem of medical-induced benzodiazepine drug dependency that continues to affect millions of unsuspecting, innocent people worldwide — either directly or indirectly.

Discussion Groups

BenzoBuddies Forum
www.benzobuddies.org/forum
By registering with the BenzoBuddies community, you will gain full access to the discussion boards; non-members participate on a read-only basis. In addition to the core parts of the community forum, there are off-topic boards, a chatroom for real-time communication, a PM (Personal Message) system for private communication and a Shoutbox (an informal short message system that displays to the whole forum). There is even an arcade to serve as a distraction during the withdrawal process.

Benzodiazepine Recovery
www.facebook.com/groups/benzorecovery
This is a discussion group for people dealing with benzodiazepine dependence and withdrawal. This group wants to spread the word on benzodiazepine withdrawal syndrome and help others heal.

Blazing Benzos
www.facebook.com/groups/1205287192817668
This page is for people who wish to discuss the benefits & pitfalls of using cannabis during benzodiazepine withdrawal and in everyday life.

Notes

Preface

[1] Frances, "Yes, Benzos Are Bad."

Introduction

[2] Ashton, *The Ashton Manual.*

[3] *Ferris Bueller's Day Off.*

[4] Ashton, *The Ashton Manual.*

Chapter 1

[5] CDC, "Leading Causes."

[6] Sommers, Jack, "Masculinity Audit into Causes of Suicide Reveals Men Suffer Depression in a Way Even Doctors Could Miss," *Huffington Post UK*, November 17, 2016, accessed April 26, 2018, https://www.huffingtonpost.co.uk/entry/mens-mental-health-building-modern-men_uk_58206805e4b0c2e24ab022fb.

[7] Kierkegaard, *The Concept of Anxiety*, 155-6 as quoted in Stossel, *My Age of Anxiety*, 3.

[8] Barlow, *Anxiety and Its Disorders,* 18.

[9] APA, *DSM-IV-TR*, 429-30.

[10] Stossel, *My Age of Anxiety*, 141.

[11] Morgan et al., "Relationship Among Plasma Cortisol."

[12] Laufer, Israeli and Paz, "Behavioral and Neural Mechanisms," 713-4.

[13] Stossel, *My Age of Anxiety*, 264.

[14] Leclerq, Forsythe and Bienenstock, "Posttraumatic Stress Disorder," 204-5.

[15] Duffie, Warren, "Gut Feeling: ONR Research Examines Link Between Stomach Bacteria, PTSD," *Navy News Service*, April 26, 2016, accessed July 1, 2018, http://www.navy.mil/submit/display.asp?story_id=94393.

[16] Stossel, *My Age of Anxiety,* 320-2.

[17] Stossel, *My Age of Anxiety,* 133-5.

18 Scutti, Susan, "Michael Phelps: 'I Am Extremely Thankful that I Did Not Take My Life'," *CNN*, January 20, 2018, accessed January 22, 2018, https://www.cnn.com/2018/01/19/health/michael-phelps-depression/index.html.

19 Shantideva, *Bodhisattva's Way of Life*, 49.

20 WHO, *Depression,* 10.

21 WHO, *Mental Health.*

22 IMS Health Data, "National Disease & Therapeutic Index: Diagnosis Visits 2002-2006," as quoted in Stossel, *My Age of Anxiety*, 300.

23 Donnelly, Laura and James Clayton, "Anxiety Disorders Have Soared Since Credit Crunch," *Telegraph*, January 1, 2012, accessed April 8, 2017, https://www.telegraph.co.uk/news/health/news/8986320/Anxiety-disorders-have-soared-since-credit-crunch.html.

24 Heitler, Susan, "The Disturbing Truth About Anxiety and Depression in College," *Psychology Today*, March 20, 2016, accessed March 7, 2017, https://www.psychologytoday.com/us/blog/resolution-not-conflict/201603/the-disturbing-truth-about-anxiety-and-depression-in-college.

25 Lewis, Katherine Reynolds, "America's Youngest Workers May Be the Least Stable Generation on Record," *Fortune*, April 28, 2016, accessed on March 7, 2017, http://fortune.com/2016/04/28/young-workers-anxiety-depression.

26 Leahy, Robert L., "How Big a Problem Is Anxiety?," *Psychology Today*, April 30, 2008, accessed June 18, 2016, https://www.psychologytoday.com/us/blog/anxiety-files/200804/how-big-problem-is-anxiety.

27 Heitler, "The Disturbing Truth."

28 Garfinkel, Renee, "Over-Anxious Americans," *Washington Times*, June 26, 2017, accessed July 5, 2017, https://www.washingtontimes.com/news/2017/jun/26/america-anxiety-disorder/.

29 WHO, *Depression*, 10.

30 Garfinkel, "Over-Anxious Americans."

31 Pew Research Center, "Social Media Fact Sheet."

32 Pea et al., "Media Use."

33 Campaign Against Living Miserably (CALM).

34 Sommers, "Masculinity Audit."

35 "How to Spot Depression in Men," *GQ,* April 19, 2016, accessed February 2, 2017, http://www.gq-magazine.co.uk/article/depression-symptoms-men.

36 Shahly, Burglund and Coulouvrat, "The Associations of Insomnia."

37 Hirshkowitz, "Sleep Time Duration."

38 Hammerschlag, "Genome-Wide Association."

39 Cho et al., "Dorsal Raphe Dopamine."

Chapter 2

40 IMS Health, *VONA.*

41 Bachhuber, Hennessy, Cunningham and Starrels, "Increasing Benzodiazepine Prescriptions."

42 Edwards, Elaine, "Bad Side-Effects of Drugs Such as Valium A 'Medical Disaster'," *Irish Times*, October 10, 2016, Accessed October 10, 2016, https://www.irishtimes.com/news/health/bad-side-effects-of-drugs-such-as-valium-a-medical-disaster-1.2824495.

43 Commonwealth of Pennsyvlania, *Prescribing Guidelines.*

44 Ashton, *The Ashton Manual.*

45 Fisher, Lawrence M., "The Happiness Quest," *Korn Ferry Institute*, August 11, 2014, accessed March 7, 2017, https://www.kornferry.com/institute/happiness-quest.

46 *Wikipedia*, "Leo Sternbach," last modified February 23, 2018, accessed April 7, 2018, https://en.wikipedia.org/wiki/Leo_Sternbach.

47 *Wikipedia*, "Leo Sternbach."

48 Stossel, *My Age of Anxiety*, 192-93.

49 Stossel, *My Age of Anxiety*, 192-93.

50 Dokoupil, Tony, "America's Long Love Affair with Anti-Anxiety Drugs," *Newsweek*, January 21, 2009, Accessed March 4, 2017, http://www.newsweek.com/americas-long-love-affair-anti-anxiety-drugs-77967.

51 Stossel, *My Age of Anxiety*, 192-193.

52 Byrne, "Benzodiazepines: The End of a Dream."

53 Stossel, *My Age of Anxiety*, 192-193.

54 *Wikipedia,* "Diazepam," last modified March 29, 2018, accessed April 7, 2018, https://en.wikipedia.org/wiki/Diazepam.

55 Ashton, "The Bridge Project."

56 Stossel, *My Age of Anxiety*, 195.

57 Balestra, Katie, "Critics Cite Serious Side Effects of Benzodiazepine Antidepressants," *Washington Post*, June 30, 2009, accessed April 7, 2018, http://www.washingtonpost.com/wp-dyn/content/article/2009/06/29/AR2009062903105.html.

58 Ashton, "The Bridge Project."

59 Bachhuber, Hennessy, Cunningham and Starrels, "Increasing Benzodiazepine Prescriptions."

60 "Global General Anxiety Disorder Market Worth USD 3,775 Million and CAGR 2.4% by 2021," *Zion Market Research*, November 18, 2016, Accessed November 19, 2016, http://www.medgadget.com/2016/11/global-general-anxiety-disorder-market-worth-usd-3775-million-and-cagr-2-4-by-2021.html.

61 Bachhumber, Hennessy, Cunningham, and Starrels, "Increasing Benzodiazepine Prescriptions."

62 IMS Health, *VONA.*

63 IMS Health, *VONA.*

64 IMS Health, *VONA.*

65 Ornstein, Charles and Ryann Grochowski Jones, "One Nation, Under Sedation: Medicare Paid for Nearly 40 Million Tranquilizer Prescriptions in 2013," *Huntington News*, February 27, 2017, accessed February 28, 2017, http://www.huntingtonnews.net/146657.

66 Barrow, Martin, "Scandal of 1 Million Caught in Tranquiliser Trap," *The Times (UK)*, October 1, 2012, accessed March 1, 2017, https://www.thetimes.co.uk/article/scandal-of-1m-caught-in-tranquilliser-trap-2glq2f0w5pr.

67 BMA, "Supporting Individuals Affected."

68 Edwards, "Bad Side-Effects."

69 Kissinger, Meg, "Thousands Prescribed Too Much Medicine," *Milwaukee Journal Sentinel*, March 15, 2017, accessed March 16, 2017, https://projects.jsonline.com/news/2017/3/15/thousands-prescribed-too-much-medicine.html.

70 Frances, "Yes, Benzos are Bad."

71 Vertosick, *When the Air*, 12.

72 Ashton, *The Ashton Manual.*

73 *Wikipedia*, "Benzodiazepine," last modified March 26, 2018, accessed April 6, 2018, https://en.wikipedia.org/wiki/Benzodiazepine.

74 NSW, "Benzodiazepines."

75 Leigh, Jennifer, "Five (5) Facts About Benzodiazepine Withdrawal (You Need to Know)," *Additionblog.org*, August 16, 2015, accessed March 6, 2017, http://prescription-drug.addictionblog.org/five-5-facts-about-benzodiazepine-withdrawal-you-need-to-know.

76 Ashton, *The Ashton Manual.*

77 *Wikipedia*, "Benzodiazepine Withdrawal Syndrome," last modified February 21, 2018, accessed April 7, 2018, https://en.wikipedia.org/wiki/Benzodiazepine_withdrawal_syndrome.

78 Ashton, *The Ashton Manual.*

79 Ashton, "Protracted Withdrawal Syndromes."

80 Ashton, "Protracted Withdrawal Syndromes."

81 "What is Dopamine?," *Psychology Today*, accessed August 10, 2017, https://www.psychologytoday.com/us/basics/dopamine.

82 NIDA, "Well-Known Mechanism."

83 Tan et al., "Neural Bases."

84 NIDA, "Well-Known Mechanism."

[85]   NIDA, "Well-Known Mechanism."

[86]   NIDA, "Well-Known Mechanism."

[87]   Ashton, *The Ashton Manual.*

[88]   "Benzodiazepine Withdrawal Support: Substitution."

Chapter 3

[89]   Fances, "Yes, Benzos are Bad."

[90]   Ramster et al., "A Policy on Benzodiazepines."

[91]   Ashton, "The Still Unfinished Story."

[92]   *Wikipedia*, "Benzodiazepine."

[93]   Porter, Mark, "Addicted to Sleeping Pills? Try This Instead," *The Sunday Times*, October 25, 2016, accessed March 4, 2017, https://www.thetimes.co.uk/article/dr-mark-porter-how-to-avoid-sleeping-tablet-addiction-shsrnpwsm.

[94]   Ashton, "Guidelines."

[95]   DEA, *Benzodiazepines.*

[96]   Commonwealth of Pennsylvania, *Prescribing Guidelines.*

[97]   NYC DOHMH, *Judicious Prescribing of Benzodiazepines.*

[98]   Bachhuber, Hennessy, Cunningham and Starrels, "Increasing Benzodiazepine Prescriptions."

[99]   Frances, "Yes, Benzos are Bad."

[100] Kripke, "Hypnotics' Association with Mortality."

[101] Ashton, "The Still Unfinished Story."

[102] Ashton, *The Ashton Manual.*

[103] Clary, Mike and Adam Sacasa, "Tiger Woods Was 'Asleep at the Wheel,' Thought He Had Been Golfing in California, DUI Report Says," *SunSentinel*, May 30, 2017, accessed June 14, 2017, http://www.sun-sentinel.com/local/palm-beach/fl-pn-tiger-woods-arrest-folo-20170530-story.html.

[104] Rayman, Graham, "Tiger Woods Tells Florida Cop He Was Taking Xanax and Vicodin Following DUI Arrest: Report," *NY Daily News*, June 10, 2017, accessed June 14, 2017, http://www.nydailynews.com/sports/more-sports/tiger-woods-tells-fla-xanax-dui-arrest-report-article-1.3236042.

[105] Oster et al., "Benzodiazepine Tranquilizers."

[106] Barker, Greenwood, Jackson and Crowe, "Cognitive Effects."

[107] Hunt, Liz and Glenn Frankel, "Britain Takes Halcion Sleeping Pills off the Market," *Washington Post*, October 3, 1991, accessed April 8, 2018, https://www.washingtonpost.com/archive/politics/1991/10/03/britain-takes-halcion-sleeping-pills-off-the-market/21d83dc2-2260-440d-96d1-7da13ceb0198/?utm_term=.e008daa4566c.

108 VA/DoD, *Use of Benzodiazepines for PTSD.*

109 Hunt and Frankel, "Britain Takes Halcion."

110 DiMascio, "Psychotropic Drugs."

111 Ashton, "Anything for a Quiet Life?"

112 Albrecht et al., "Benzodiazepine Use."

113 Pink Floyd, *Comfortably Numb.*

114 Ashton, *The Ashton Manual.*

115 Cox, Lauren, "Tranquilizer Detox Withdrawal Can Last Years," *ABC News*, December 1, 2008, accessed January 30, 2017, http://abcnews.go.com/Health/DepressionNews/story?id=6354685&page=1.

116 Longo and Johnson, "Addiction: Part I."

117 NSW, "Benzodiazepines."

118 Ashton, *The Ashton Manual.*

119 NYC DOHMH, *Judicious Prescribing of Benzodiazepines*, 16.

120 NHS, "Guidance for Prescribing," 8.

121 Aubrey, Allison, "Benefits Can Outweigh Risks for Pregnant Women on Anxiety Drugs or SSRIs," *NPR Shots*, September 18, 2017, accessed September 18, 2017, http://www.npr.org/sections/health-shots/2017/09/18/551020800/xanax-or-zoloft-for-moms-to-be-a-new-study-assesses-safety.

122 Doyle, Chase, "Benzodiazepine Exposure Can Predict Delirium in Critically Ill Children," *Anesthesiology News*, October 13, 2016, accessed October 13, 2016, http://www.anesthesiologynews.com/Clinical-Anesthesiology/Article/10-16/Benzodiazepine-Exposure-Can-Predict-Delirium-in-Critically-Ill-Children/38055.

123 Frances, "Yes, Benzos Are Bad."

124 Commonwealth of Pennsylvania, *Prescribing Guidelines.*

125 Ashton, *The Ashton Manual.*

126 Saarelainen et al., "Risk of death."

127 Frances, "Yes, Benzos Are Bad."

128 Billioti de Gage et al., "Benzodiazepine Use and Risk."

129 Pariente, Billioti de Gage, Moore and Bégaud, "The Benzodiazepine-Dementia Disorders Link."

130 Pariente, Billioti de Gage, Moore and Bégaud, "The Benzodiazepine-Dementia Disorders Link."

131 NIDA, "Is There a Difference?"

132 NIDA, "Is There a Difference?"

133 NIDA, "Definition of Tolerance."

134 NIDA, "Is There a Difference?"

135   Lader, "History of Benzodiazepine Dependence."

136   "10 Most Addictive Drugs List," *Mental Health Daily*, October 10, 2014, accessed August 6, 2017, http://mentalhealthdaily.com/2014/10/10/10-most-addictive-drugs-list.

137   Ashton, *The Ashton Manual*.

138   Ashton, "Toxicity and Adverse Consequences."

139   Lane, "Brain Damage from Benzodiazepines."

140   Lakhani, Nina, "Drugs Linked to Brain Damage 30 Years Ago," *Independent*, November 7, 2010, accessed March 4, 2017, https://www.independent.co.uk/life-style/health-and-families/health-news/drugs-linked-to-brain-damage-30-years-ago-2127504.html.

141   Lane, "Brain Damage from Benzodiazepines."

142   Porter, "Addicted to Sleeping Pills?"

143   VA/DoD, *Use of Benzodiazepines for PTSD*.

Chapter 4

144   DEA, *Benzodiazepines*.

145   CDC, "Drugs Most Frequently Involved."

146   "Popping Xanax is More Harmful than You Think," *Fox News*, January 31, 2014, accessed January 31, 2014, http://www.foxnews.com/health/2014/01/31/popping-xanax-is-more-harmful-than-think.html.

147   McCain, Cilla, "Dying in their Sleep: The Invisible Plague Attacking U.S. Soldiers," *HuffPost*, June 23, 2010, updated December 6, 2017, accessed April 9, 2018, https://www.huffingtonpost.com/cilla-mccain/dying-in-their-sleep-the_b_618429.html.

148   NYC DOHMH, *Judicious Prescribing of Benzodiazepines*, 15.

149   Storrs, Carina, "Benzodiazepine Overdose Deaths Soared in Recent Years, Study Finds," *CNN*, updated February 18, 2016, accessed January 30, 2017, https://www.cnn.com/2016/02/18/health/benzodiazepine-sedative-overdose-death-increase/index.html.

150   "Popping Xanax," *Fox News*.

151   "Popping Xanax," *Fox News*.

152   Hawryluk, Markian, "Benzodiazepines Treat Anxiety, Vause long-term problems," *Bend Bulletin*, June 1, 2014, updated June 3, 2014, accessed January 30, 2017, http://www.bendbulletin.com/localstate/2119922-151/benzodiazepines-treat-anxiety-cause-long-term-problems#.

153   Huxley, *Brave New World*.

154   Frances, "Yes, Benzos are Bad."

155 Maust et al., "No End in Sight."
156 Maust et al., "No End in Sight."
157 AGS, "Updated Beers Criteria."
158 IMS Health, *VONA*.
159 Kim and Weinstein, "Johns Hopkins Psychiatry Guide."

Chapter 5

160 Rolling Stones, *Mother's Little Helper*.
161 Reed, *Walk on the Wild Side*.
162 Costello, *This Year's Girl*.
163 The Escape Club, *Wild, Wild West*.
164 Kottke, *Big Mob on the Hill*.
165 Duran Duran, *Lady Xanax*.
166 Queens of the Stone Age, *Feel Good Hit of the Summer*.
167 Lil Wyte, *Oxy Cotton*.
168 OK Go, *A Million Ways*.
169 Lil Wayne, *I Feel Like Dying*.
170 Morrissey, *Something Is Squeezing My Skull*.
171 Mayer, *Heartbreak Warfare*.
172 Jay-Z and Keys, *Empire State of Mind*.
173 Pill Friends, *Klonopin*.
174 Halsey, *Colours*.
175 blink-182, *Wildfire*.
176 Drake, *Two Birds, One Stone*.
177 Arcade Fire, *Put Your Money on Me*.
178 *Starting Over*.
179 *Fight Club*.
180 *American Psycho*.
181 *28 Days Later*.
182 *The Hours*.
183 *The Simpsons*, "Crook and Ladder."
184 *The Big Bang Theory*, "The Bad Fish Paradigm."
185 *Fringe*, "Unearthed."
186 *Bridesmaids*.

[187] *Silver Linings Playbook.*

[188] *The Late Show Starring Stephen Colbert*, Season 2, Episode 108.

[189] McKay, Hollie, "Stevie Nicks Says Doc Almost Killed Her, Ruined Chance of Becoming a Mom," *Fox News*, May 4, 2011, accessed December 12, 2016, http://www.foxnews.com/entertainment/2011/05/04/exclusive-stevie-nicks-says-doc-killed-ruined-chance-mom.html.

[190] Byron, Christopher, "The Deadliest Prescription Drug in America?," *The Fix*, February 9, 2015, accessed June 20, 2017, https://www.thefix.com/content/worlds-most-dangerous-drug?page=all.

[191] Coleman, Miriam, "Chris Brown Suffers from Bipolar Disorder, PTSD, Says Court Report," *Rolling Stone*, March 1, 2014, accessed March 3, 2017, https://www.rollingstone.com/music/news/chris-brown-suffers-from-bipolar-disorder-ptsd-says-court-report-20140301.

[192] Fleischer, Adam, "Chris Brown Opens Up About How Lean and Xanax Hurt His Productivity," *MTV.com*, October 31, 2014, accessed March 3, 2017, http://www.mtv.com/news/1983036/chris-opens-up-about-how-lean-and-xanax-hurt-his-productivity.

[193] Farrand, Stephen, "Paolini Abandons Hope of a Comeback After Serving Ban for Cocaine," *Cycling News*, January 18, 2017, accessed January 19, 2017, http://www.cyclingnews.com/news/paolini-abandons-hope-of-a-comeback-after-serving-ban-for-cocaine.

[194] Hedegaard, Erik, "The Dirty Mind and Lonely Heart of John Mayer," *Rolling Stone*, June 6, 2012, January 19, 2016, https://www.rollingstone.com/music/news/the-dirty-mind-and-lonely-heart-of-john-mayer-20120606?page=2.

[195] "K-Pop Superstar T.O.P. in Intensive Care After Overdose," *BBC News*, June 8, 2017, accessed June 14, 2017, http://www.bbc.com/news/world-asia-40199562.

[196] Goldman, Russell, "Elvis Presley's Death: Anniversary Spotlights Similarities with Michael Jackson," *ABC News*, August 16, 2009, accessed April 26, 2018, https://abcnews.go.com/Entertainment/story?id=8331541&page=1.

[197] Byron, Christopher, "Is This the World's Deadliest Pill?," *The Fix*, May 22, 2011, accessed April 9, 2018, https://www.thefix.com/content/worlds-most-dangerous-drug?page=all.

[198] Childs, Dan, "Anna Nicole Smith's Overdose — a Prescription for Death," *ABC News*, March 26, 2007, accessed April 9, 2018, http://abcnews.go.com/Health/story?id=2982443&page=1.

[199] "Ledger's Death Caused by Accidental Overdose," *CNN*, February 6, 2008, accessed April 9, 2018, http://www.cnn.com/2008/SHOWBIZ/Movies/02/06/heath.ledger.

[200] "The Drugs Found in Michael Jackson's Body After He Died," *BBC*, November 8, 2011, accessed April 9, 2018, http://www.bbc.co.uk/newsbeat/article/15634083/the-drugs-found-in-michael-jacksons-body-after-he-died.

201 Newman, Jason, "Chris Cornell's Widow: 'Several Unanswered Questions' About Singer's Suicide," *Rolling Stone*, June 1, 2017, accessed June 14, 2017, https://www.rollingstone.com/music/news/chris-cornells-widow-i-have-several-unanswered-questions-w485181.

202 Kreps, Daniel, "Chris Cornell Autopsy Report: 'Drugs Did Not Contribute' to Death," *Rolling Stone*, June 2, 2017, accessed June 14, 2017, https://www.rollingstone.com/music/news/chris-cornell-autopsy-and-toxicology-report-released-w484309.

203 "CCHR: Another Celebrity Lost to Benzodiazepines and Opioids Mix," *PR Neswire*, January 25, 2018, accessed January 26, 2018, http://markets.businessinsider.com/news/stocks/cchr-another-celebrity-lost-to-benzodiazepines-and-opioids-mix-1013996762.

204 Grow, Kory, "Lil Peep Cause of Death Revealed," *Rolling Stone*, December 8, 2017, accessed April 9, 2018, https://www.rollingstone.com/music/news/lil-peep-cause-of-death-revealed-w513699.

205 Lil Peep, *Praying to the Sky.*

Chapter 6

206 ITA, *2016 Top Markets Report.*

207 Melin, Anders, "If You Want to Be a Rich CEO, Work in Health Care," *Bloomberg*, January 6, 2017, accessed January 6, 2017, https://www.bloomberg.com/news/articles/2017-01-06/the-highest-paid-u-s-executives-supervise-doctors-not-bankers?cmpid=flipboard.

208 Ventola, "Direct-to-Consumer."

209 Ventola, "Direct-to-Consumer."

210 Horovitz, Bruce and Julie Appleby, "Pharma TV Ad Spend Promoting Prescription Drugs Has Increased 62 Percent Since 2012," *MedCity News*, March 20, 2017, Accessed April 8, 2017, https://medcitynews.com/2017/03/pharma-tv-ad-spend-promoting-prescription-drugs.

211 Ashton, "The Bridge Project."

212 Dokoupil, Tony, "America's Long Love Affair."

213 Horovitz and Appleby, "Pharma TV Ad Spend."

214 Hawryluk, "Benzodiazepines Treat Anxiety."

215 Allan, Angela, "How the 'Evil Corporation' Became a Pop-Culture Trope," *The Atlantic*, April 25, 2016, accessed February 16, 2017, https://www.theatlantic.com/business/archive/2016/04/evil-corporation-trope/479295.

216 Downing et al., "Postmarket Safety Events."

217 DEA, *Drug Scheduling.*

218 Ashton, "The Bridge Project."

219 Lader, "History of Benzodiazepine Dependence."

220 DH, *Benzodiazepines Warning.*

221 NHS, "Guidance for Prescribing."

222 NICE, "Pharmacological Treatment."

223 O'Keeffe, Cormac, "Laws Tackle Booming Trade in Sedatives and Sleeping Tablets," *Irish Examiner*, May 5, 2017, accessed June 14, 2017, https://www.irishexaminer.com/ireland/laws-tackle-booming-trade-in-sedatives-and-sleeping-tablets-449407.html.

224 FDA, "FDA Requires Strong Warnings."

225 Commonwealth of Pennsylvania, *Prescribing Guidelines.*

226 Commonwealth of Massachusetts, *Bill H.3594.*

227 NYC DOHMH, *Judicious Prescribing of Benzodiazepines.*

228 CPSA, "Check-Up for Benzodiazepine."

229 MCHK, Guidelines on the Proper Prescription.

230 Chung, "Benzodiazepine Prescribing Trend."

231 Lakhani, Nina. "Check on Benzodiazepine-Use Must Be Done, Say MPs," *The Independent*, December 5, 2010, accessed March 6, 2017, https://www.independent.co.uk/life-style/health-and-families/health-news/check-on-benzodiazepine-use-must-be-done-say-mps-2151707.html.

Chapter 7

232 King, "Is There Still a Role."

233 White, Caroline. "Be Careful When Prescribing Benzodiazepines, Doctors Warned," *OnMedica*, October 26, 2016, accessed October 26, 2016, http://www.onmedica.com/newsArticle.aspx?id=bc9d74e2-4bd2-4792-b1d3-e154f4fe4bb5.

234 Lakhani, "Drugs Linked to Brain Damage."

235 Waters, Jo, "Why Are 250,000 Lives Still Being Ruined by Mother's Little Helpers? Doctors Finally Admit Too Many Patients Are Hooked on Tranquilisers," *Daily Mail*, November 7, 2016, accessed December 22, 2016, http://www.dailymail.co.uk/health/article-3915114/Why-250-000-lives-ruined-mother-s-little-helpers-Doctors-finally-admit-patients-hooked-tranquilisers.html#.

236 Waters, "Why Are 250,000 Lives."

237 Lakhani, "Drugs Linked to Brain Damage."

238 Lakhani, "Drugs Linked to Brain Damage."

239 Matott, Sarah, "John Patrick Walter Attorneys: Provider Had 'Money-Making' Motive," *Cañon Cityy News*, March 6, 2017, accessed April 11,2018, http://www.canoncitydailyrecord.com/news/canoncity-local-news/ci_30839522/john-patrick-walter-attorneys-provider-had-money-making.

240 Roberts, Michael, "'Atrocity': The Agonizing, Unnecessary, 18-Day Jail Death of John Patrick Walter," *Westword*, January 25, 2017, accessed January 25, 2017, http://www.westword.com/news/atrocity-the-agonizing-unnecessary-18-day-jail-death-of-john-patrick-walter-8688441.

241 Benzel, Lance, "Cause-of-Death Finding Bolsters Cover-Up Claim in Fremont County Jail Inmate's Death," *The Colorado Springs Gazette*, May 14, 2017, updated May 15, 2017, accessed August 24, 2017, http://gazette.com/cause-of-death-finding-bolsters-cover-up-claim-in-fremont-county-jail-inmates-death/article/1603116.

242 Benzel, "Cause-of-Death."

243 Benzel, "Cause-of-Death."

244 Roberts, "Atrocity."

245 Benzel, "Cause-of-Death."

246 Matott, "John Patrick Walter."

247 Benzel, "Cause-of-Death."

248 Flynn, Meagan, "Jesse Jacobs Died in Lockup Six Days After Galveston County Jailers Cut Off His Meds," *Houston Press*, August 6, 2015, April 10, 2018, http://www.houstonpress.com/news/jesse-jacobs-died-in-lockup-six-days-after-galveston-county-jailers-cut-off-his-meds-7646761.

249 Lopez, German, "David Stojcevski's Horrifying Death in Jail, Explained," *Vox*, updated September 29, 2015, accessed April 10, 2018, https://www.vox.com/2015/9/26/9399391/macomb-county-jail-david-stojcevski.

250 Hall, Christina, "U.S. Attorney Says Evidence in David Stojcevski's Death Doesn't Support Criminal Civil Rights Violation Charges," *Detroit Free Press*, September 19, 2016, accessed April 10, 2018, https://www.freep.com/story/news/local/michigan/macomb/2016/09/19/macomb-jail-death-inmate-david-stojcevski/90688274.

251 Board of Cuyahoga County, *Sean's Law Briefing.*

252 Miller, Donna J., "Sean Levert, Denied Medication, Hallucinated for Hours Before He Died in Jail," *The Plain Dealer*, November 11, 2008, accessed April 10, 2018, http://blog.cleveland.com/metro/2008/11/post_15.html.

Chapter 8

253 Ashton, *The Ashton Manual.*

254 Lindskog, "Pharmaceutical Residue in Water."

255 Arnnok et al., "Selective Uptake and Bioaccumulation."

256   "Study Finds Traces of Drugs in Drinking Water in 24 Major U.S. Regions," *Fox News / AP,* March 10, 2008, accessed March 6, 2017, http://www.foxnews.com/story/2008/03/10/study-finds-traces-drugs-in-drinking-water-in-24-major-us-regions.html.

257   Ben-Ami Bartal et al., "Anxiolytic Treatment Impairs."

258   Lader, Malcolm, *BBC Interview,* 1999 as quoted in Lane, Christopher, "Brain Damage from Benzodiazepines."

259   "Professor Malcolm H Lader," *BenzoBuddies.*

260   Ashton, *The Ashton Manual.*

261   "About W-BAD."

262   Ashton, *The Ashton Manual.*

263   Ashton, *The Ashton Manual.*

264   Lakhani, "Drugs Linked to Brain Damage."

265   Ashton, *The Ashton Manual.*.

266   Frances, "Yes, Benzos Are Bad."

267   *Wikipedia,* "Allen Frances," last modified September 8, 2017, accessed October 13, 2017, https://en.wikipedia.org/wiki/Allen_Frances.

268   Frances, "Yes, Benzos Are Bad."

269   Osmond, Michelle, "Safe Prescribing: Faculty of Medicine Addressing Opioid Abuse in N.L.," *University Memorial Gazette,* March 3, 2017, accessed March 4, 2017, https://gazette.mun.ca/teaching-and-learning/safe-prescribing.

270   Forde, Emma, "Doctors' Leaders Call for Prescription Drug Helpline," *BBC News,* October 23, 2016, accessed October 24, 2016, http://www.bbc.com/news/health-37716869.

Chapter 9

271   Trickett, "Withdrawal from Benzodiazepines."

272   Byrne, "Benzodiazepines: The End of a Dream."

273   Maletzky and Klotter, "Addiction to Diazepam."

274   Naish, John, "Betrayed by the Doctors Who Turned Us into DRUG ADDICTS: How a Nation of Patients Became Hooked on Prescription Pills," *Daily Mail,* May 22, 2017, accessed June 14, 2017, http://www.dailymail.co.uk/health/article-4531548/Betrayed-doctors-turned-DRUG-ADDICTS.html.

275   Ashton, "The Bridge Project."

276   Lader, "Limitations on the Use."

277 Bleyer, Jennifer, "Popping Xanax Is More Harmful Than You Think," *Self*, February 20, 2014, accessed January 30, 2017, https://www.self.com/story/xanax-more-harmful-than-you-think.

278 Frances, "Yes, Benzos are Bad."

279 Hawryluk, "Benzodiazepines Treat Anxiety."

280 NYC DOHMH, *Judicious Prescribing of Benzodiazepines*, 14.

281 Ashton, "The Bridge Project."

282 DH, *Benzodiazepines Warning*.

283 NHS, "Guidance for Prescribing."

284 *Benzodiazepine Medical Disaster*, RTÉ Ireland.

285 Forde, "Doctors' Leaders Call."

286 *Face the Facts*, "Prescribed Addiction."

287 Pétursson, "The Benzodiazepine Withdrawal Syndrome."

288 Cox, "Tranquilizer Detox Withdrawal."

289 Fox, "When Withdrawal."

290 *In Pills We Trust,* Discovery Channel.

291 Smith, "Sleeping Pills Overprescribed."

292 Rickels, Case, Downing, and Winokur, "Long-Term Diazepam Therapy."

293 Ashton, "The Still Unfinished Story."

294 Higgitt, Fonagy, Toone, and Shine, "The Prolonged Benzodiazepine Withdrawal."

295 Lader and Morton, "A Pilot Study."

296 *The Tranquilisers Trap*, BBC-1.

297 Olfson, King and Schoenbaum, "Benzodiazepine Use in the United States."

298 Lakhani, "Check on Benzodiazepine-Use."

Chapter 10

299 Keefer, Brooke, "The Nightmare of Benzodiazepine Withdrawal," *Hormones Matter,* May 23, 2017, accessed March 6, 2017, http://www.hormonesmatter.com/nightmare-benzodiazepine-withdrawal.

300 Kenny, Shane, "Tranquillisers drove me to the brink of suicide," *The Sunday Times*, October 9, 2016, accessed March 4, 2017, https://www.thetimes.co.uk/article/tranquillisers-drove-me-to-the-brink-of-suicide-z23npq76r.

301 Cox, "Tranquilizer Detox Withdrawal."

302 *The Tranquilisers Trap*, BBC-1.

303 *The Tranquilisers Trap*, BBC-1.

[304] Fox, "When Withdrawal Is the Hardest Part."

[305] *The Tranquilisers Trap*, BBC-1.

[306] Naish, "Betrayed by the Doctors."

[307] Ashton, *The Ashton Manual.*

Chapter 11

[308] *Wikipedia*, "Benzodiazepine Withdrawal Syndrome."

[309] Ashton, "Protracted Withdrawal Syndromes."

[310] Ashton, "Protracted Withdrawal Syndromes."

[311] Higgitt, Lader and Fonagy, "Clinical Management."

[312] Ashton, "Toxicity and Adverse Consequences."

[313] *Face the Facts*, "Prescribed Addiction."

[314] Liebrenz, Gehring, Buadze and Caflisch, "High-Dose Benzodiazepine Dependence."

[315] Pétursson and Lader, "Withdrawal from Long-Term Benzodiazepine."

[316] Ashton, "Post-Withdrawal Syndrome."

[317] Ashton, "Post-Withdrawal Syndrome."

[318] Javed, "Misuse of Benzodiazepine."

[319] "Protracted Withdrawal Syndrome (PWS)," W-BAD.

[320] Maletzky and Klotter, "Addiction to Diazepam."

[321] Ashton, "Protracted Withdrawal from Benzodiazepines."

[322] Ashton, *The Ashton Manual.*

[323] *Merriam-Webster* (online), "Taper," accessed January 20, 2018, https://www.merriam-webster.com/dictionary/taper.

[324] Ashton, *The Ashton Manual.*

[325] "Direct Tapers."

[326] Ashton, *The Ashton Manual.*

[327] Ashton, *The Ashton Manual.*

[328] Ashton, *The Ashton Manual* and "Benzodiazepine Withdrawal Methods," *Benzo Buddies.*

Chapter 12

[329] Ashton, *The Ashton Manual.*

330   Multiple Sources: Ashton, *The Ashton Manual,* "Benzodiazepine Withdrawal Support," *Wikipedia* (varied).

331   "About ADAA: Facts & Statistics."

332   "About ADAA: Facts & Statistics."

333   Ashton, *The Ashton Manual.*

334   Donnelly, Laura, "'Cyberchondria' Fuelling Anxiety Epidemic Clogging Up Hospital Clinics," *The Telegraph,* September 7, 2017, accessed September 8, 2017, https://www.telegraph.co.uk/news/2017/09/07/cyberchondria-fuelling-anxiety-epidemic-clogging-hospital-clinics.

335   Manson, *The Subtle Art,* 117.

336   Gorenstein, Bernik and Pompéia, "Differential Acute Psychomotor."

337   Tata et al., "Lack of Cognitive Recovery."

338   Ashton, *The Ashton Manual.*

339   Ashton, *The Ashton Manual.*

340   "Depersonalization-Derealization Disorder," Mayo Clinic.

341   "Overview of Sleep Disorders," *Harvard Medical School.*

342   Ashton, *The Ashton Manual.*

343   APA, *DSM-IV-TR.*

344   Multiple Sources: Ashton, *The Ashton Manual,* "Benzodiazepine Withdrawal Support," *Wikipedia* (varied).

345   Ashton, *The Ashton Manual*

346   Ashton, *The Ashton Manual.*

Chapter 13

347   Ashton, *The Ashton Manual.*

348   Ashton, *The Ashton Manual.*

349   Ashton, *The Ashton Manual.*

350   Ashton, *The Ashton Manual.*

351   Bach, *Illusions,* 75.

352   Meixler, Eli, "'Remember to Look Up at the Stars.' Read Some of Stephen Hawking's Most Memorable Quotes," *Time,* March 14, 2018, accessed March 15, 2018, http://time.com/5198842/stephen-hawking-quotes-universe-life.

353   Roser and Ortiz-Ospina, "Global Rise of Education."

354   Roser and Ortiz-Ospina, "Global Extreme Poverty."

355   Roser and Ortiz-Ospina, "Homicides."

356   McCarthy, "More Americans Say Crime."

357 *Finding Nemo.*

358 Babyak et al., "Exercise Treatment for Major Depression."

359 Ashton, *The Ashton Manual.*

Chapter 14

360 Ashton, *The Ashton Manual.*

361 Ashton, *The Ashton Manual.*

362 Ashton, *The Ashton Manual.*

363 Ashton, *The Ashton Manual.*

364 "Frequently Asked Questions," *BenzoBuddies,* accessed March 1, 2017, http://www.benzobuddies.org/benzodiazepine-information/frequently-asked-questions.

365 Ashton, *The Ashton Manual.*

366 Ashton, *The Ashton Manual.*

367 Ashton, *The Ashton Manual.*

368 Ashton, *The Ashton Manual.*

369 "Frequently Asked Questions," *BenzoBuddies.*

370 Ashton, *The Ashton Manual.*

371 FDA, "FDA Drug Safety."

372 Ashton, *The Ashton Manual.*

373 Lader and Morton, "A Pilot Study."

374 Ashton, *The Ashton Manual.*

375 Ashton, *The Ashton Manual.*

376 WHO, "Cannabidiol (CBD)."

Chapter 15

377 Gibran, *The Prophet*, 60.

Chapter 17

378 Dickens, *Great Expectations*, 185.

Appendix

379 Multiple Sources:
   Ashton, *The Ashton Manual,*
   "Benzodiazepine Withdrawal Support: Substitution," Benzo Buddies,
   "Generic Benzodiazepines and Brand," Benzo Buddies,
   Government of South Australia, "Benzodiazepine Equivalents,"
   NHS, "Guidance for Prescribing,"
   "PubChem Open Chemistry Database," NIH,
   Wikipedia (varied).

Bibliography

28 Days Later. Directed by Danny Boyle. Los Angeles: Twentieth Century Fox, 2002.

"About ADAA: Facts & Statistics." Anxiety and Depression Association of America. Accessed February 24, 2018. https://adaa.org/about-adaa/press-room/facts-statistics#.

"About the Associative Awareness Techniques (AAT) Program." Wellness & Performance. Accessed March 23, 2018. http://www.wellnessandperformance.com/about.html.

"About W-BAD." World Benzodiazepine Awareness Day (WBAD). Accessed April 11, 2018. http://w-bad.org/about/.

Albrecht, Bonnie, Petra K. Staiger, Kate Hall, Peter Miller, David Best and Dan I. Lubman. "Benzodiazepine Use and Aggressive Behaviour: A Systematic Review." *Australian & New Zealand Journal of Psychiatry* 48(12)(September 2, 2014):1096-114. Accessed April 16, 2018. doi:10.1177/0004867414548902.

American Geriatrics Society (AGS). "American Geriatrics Society 2015 Updated Beers Criteria for Potentially Inappropriate Medication Use in Older Adults." *Beers Criteria Update Expert Panel* (2015). Accessed April 9, 2018. http://www.sigot.org/allegato_docs/1057_Beers-Criteria.pdf.

American Psychiatric Association (APA). *Diagnostic and Statistical Manual of Mental Disorders* 4th ed. text rev. (DSM-IV-TR). Washington, DC: American Psychiatric Association, 2000.

American Psycho. Directed by Mary Harron. Los Angeles: Lionsgate, 2000.

Arcade Fire. *Put Your Money on Me.* Columbia, 2018. https://genius.com/Arcade-fire-put-your-money-on-me-lyrics.

Arnnok, Prapha, Randolph R. Singh, Rodjana Burakham, Alicia Pérez-Fuenteteja and Diana S. Aga. "Selective Uptake and Bioaccumulation of Antidepressants in Fish from Effluent-Impacted Niagara River." *Environmental Science & Technology* 51(18)(August 16, 2017):10652-62. Accessed September 7, 2017. doi:10.1021/acs.est.7b02912.

Ashton, C. Heather. "Adverse Effects of Prolonged Benzodiazepine Use." *Adverse Drug Reaction Bulletin* 118(1):440-3. Accessed April 8, 2017. https://www.benzo.org.uk/adv.htm.

———. "Anything for a Quiet Life?: Valium, Librium and Mogadon Once Seemed to Provide the Perfect Answer to Stress. We Now Know How this Group of Drugs Alters the Chemistry of the Brain; No Wonder They Create More Problems Than They Solve." *New Scientist* 6(May 1989). Accessed May 3, 2017. https://www.newscientist.com/article/mg12216635-400/.

———. *Benzodiazepines: How They Work and How to Withdraw (aka The Ashton Manual)*. 2002. Accessed April 13, 2016. http://www.benzo.org.uk/manual/.

———. "Benzodiazepines: The Still Unfinished Story." (Speech at Beat the Benzos Launch Conference, Croyden, London, England). https://www.benzo.org.uk/ashspeech.htm.

———. "Guidelines for the Rational Use of Benzodiazepines." *Drugs* 48(1) (July 1994):25-40. Accessed March 6, 2017. https://www.ncbi.nlm.nih.gov/pubmed/7525193.

———. "Protracted Withdrawal from Benzodiazepines: The Post-Withdrawal Syndrome." *Psychiatric Annals* 25(3)(1995):174-179. Accessed April 14, 2018. doi:10.3928/0048-5713-19950301-11.

———. "Protracted Withdrawal Syndromes from Benzodiazepines." *Journal of Substance Abuse Treatment* 8 (1991): 19-28. https://www.benzo.org.uk/ashpws.htm.

———. "The Bridge Project, Bradford: Speech by Professor C Heather Ashton, DM FRCP: Annual Meeting, December 2011." Benzo.org.uk. Accessed January 27, 2017. https://www.benzo.org.uk/chabradford.htm.

———. "Toxicity and Adverse Consequences of Benzodiazepine Use." *Physician Annals* 25 (March 1995):158-65. Accessed March 6, 2017. https://www.benzo.org.uk/ashtox.htm.

Babyak, Michael, James A. Blumenthal, Steve Herman, Parinda Khatri, Murali Doraiswamy, Kathleen Moore, Edward Craighead, Teri T. Baldewicz and K. Ranga Krishnan. "Exercise Treatment for Major Depression: Maintenance of Therapeutic Benefit at 10 Months." *Psychosomatic Medicine* 62(5)(October 2000):633-38. Accessed April 12, 2018. http://www.hibody.co.uk/Exercise%20treatment%20for%20major%20depression.pdf.

Bach, Richard. *Illusions: The Adventures of a Reluctant Messiah.* New York: Creature Enterprises, 1977. Print.

Bachhuber, Marcus A., Sean Hennessy, Chinazo O. Cunningham and Joanna L. Starrels. "Increasing Benzodiazepine Prescriptions and Overdose Mortality in the United States, 1996-2013." *American Journal of Public Health (AJPH)* (April 2016). Accessed April 7, 2018. doi:10.2105/AJPH.2016.303061.

Barker, M.J., K.M. Greenwood, M. Jackson, S.F. Crowe. "Cognitive Effects of Long-Term Benzodiazepine Use: A Meta-Analysis." *CNS Drugs* 18(1)(2004):37-48. Accessed March 6, 2017. https://www.ncbi.nlm.nih.gov/pubmed/14731058.

Barlow, David. *Anxiety and Its Disorders.* 2nd ed. New York: The Guilford Press, 2002.

Ben-Ami Bartal, Inbal, Haozhe Shan, Nora M. R. Molasky, Teresa M. Murray, Jasper Z. Williams, Jean Decety and Peggy Mason. "Anxiolytic Treatment Impairs Helping Behavior in Rats." *Frontiers in Psychology* 7(2016):850. Accessed March 6, 2017. doi:10.3389/fpsyg.2016.00850.

Ben-Shahar, Tal. *Happier: Learn the Secrets to Daily Joy and Lasting Fulfillment.* New York: McGraw-Hill, 2007.

Benzodiazepine Medical Disaster. RTÉ Ireland. October 2016. Directed by Shane Kenny. Quoted by Edwards, Elaine. "Bad Side-Effects of Drugs such as Valium a 'Medical Disaster.'" *Irish Times.* October 10, 2016. Accessed January 19, 2017. https://www.irishtimes.com/news/health/bad-side-effects-of-drugs-such-as-valium-a-medical-disaster-1.2824495.

"Benzodiazepine Withdrawal Support: Substitution." *BenzoBuddies*. Accessed March 1, 2017. http://www.benzobuddies.org/benzodiazepine-withdrawal-methods/substitution/.

"Benzodiazepine Withdrawal Support: Benzodiazepine Withdrawal Methods." *BenzoBuddies*. Accessed May 3, 2018. http://www.benzobuddies.org/benzodiazepine-withdrawal-methods/overview/.

Bergman, Hans, Stefan Borg, Karin Engelbrekston and Britt Vikander. "Dependence on Sedative-Hypnotics: Neuropsychological Impairment, Field Dependence and Clinical Course in a 5-Year Follow-Up Study." *British Journal of Addiction* 84(May 1989):547-53. Accessed April 15, 2018. doi:10.1111/j.1360-0443.1989.tb00612.x.

The Big Bang Theory. "The Bad Fish Paradigm." Directed by Mark Cendrowski. Written by David Goetsch, Steven Molaro, and Bill Prady. Warner Bros. Television, September 22, 2008.

Billioti de Gage, Sophie, Yola Moride, Thierry Ducruet, Tobias Kurth, Hélène Verdoux, Marie Tournier, Antoine Pariente and Bernard Bégaud. "Benzodiazepine Use and Risk of Alzheimer's Disease: Case-Control Study." *BMJ* 349(g5205)(2014). Accessed January 30, 2017. doi:10.1136/bmj.g5205.

blink-182. *Wildfire*. BMG, 2016. http://www.metrolyrics.com/wildfire-lyrics-blink-182.html.

Board of Cuyahoga County: Alcohol, Drug Addiction & Mental Health Services. *HB 84: Sean's Law Briefing*. Accessed April 10, 2018. http://adamhscc.org/en-us/seans-law-briefing.aspx.

Bowen, Will. *A Complaint Free World: How to Stop Complaining and Start Enjoying the Life You Always Wanted*. New York: Three Rivers Press, 2007.

Bridesmaids. Directed by Paul Feig. Los Angeles: Universal Pictures, 2011.

British Medical Association (BMA). "Supporting Individuals Affected by Prescribed Drugs Associated with Dependence and Withdrawal." *Our Collective Voice*. October 6, 2016. Accessed June 14, 2017. https://www.bma.org.uk/collective-voice/policy-and-research/public-and-population-health/prescribed-drugs-dependence-and-withdrawal.

Byrne, A. "Benzodiazepines: The End of a Dream." *Australian Family Physician* 23(8)(Aug 1994):1584-5. Accessed April 17, 2018. https://www.ncbi.nlm.nih.gov/pubmed/7980158.

Campaign Against Living Miserably (CALM). Home Page. Accessed April 20, 2018. https://www.thecalmzone.net/.

Canfield, Jack. "Become an Inverse Paranoid." *Jack Canfield*. Accessed September 22, 2017. http://jackcanfield.com/blog/become-an-inverse-paranoid/.

Cho, Jounhong Ryan, Jennifer B. Treweek, J. Elliott Robinson, Cheng Xiao, Lindsay R. Bremner, Alon Greenbaum and Viviana Gradinaru. "Dorsal Raphe Dopamine Neurons Modulate Arousal and Promote Wakefulness by Salient Stimuli." Abstract. *Neuron* 94(6): 1205-19. doi:10.1016/j.neuron.2017.05.020.

Chung, K.F. "Benzodiazepines Prescribing Trend After Its Inclusion as a Dangerous Drug Under the Hong Kong Dangerous Drugs Ordinance." Reprint. Hong Kong Medical Journal 3(1) (1997):16-20. Accessed April 8, 2018. https://www.benzo.org.uk/amisc/hk.pdf.

College of Physicians & Surgeons of Alberta (CPSA). "A Check-Up for Benzodiazepine Prescribing Practice." *Messenger: Prescribing Corner*. June 11, 2015. Accessed April 10, 2018. http://www.cpsa.ca/check-benzodiazepine-prescribing-practice/.

Commonwealth of Massachusetts: 190th General Court. *Bill H.3594: An Act Relative to Benzodiazepines and Non-Benzodiazepine Hypnotics*. Presented by Paul McMurtry. Accessed April 10, 2018. https://malegislature.gov/Bills/190/H3594.

Commonwealth of Pennsylvania. *Prescribing Guidelines for Pennsylvania: Safe Prescribing Benzodiazepines for Acute Treatment of Anxiety & Insomnia*. Updated May 15, 2017. Accessed April 7, 2018. http://www.health.pa.gov/My%20Health/Diseases%20and%20Conditions/M-P/opioids/Documents/PA%20Guidelines%20on%20Benzo%20Prescribing.pdf.

Costello, Elvis. *This Year's Girl*. Columbia, 1978. https://genius.com/Elvis-costello-this-years-girl-lyrics.

"Depersonalization-Derealization Disorder." Mayo Clinic. Accessed May 1, 2018. https://www.mayoclinic.org/diseases-conditions/depersonalization-derealization-disorder/diagnosis-treatment/drc-20352916.

Dickens, Charles. *Doctor Marigold*. Oxford: Oxford University Press, 2002.

Dickens, Charles. *Great Expectations*. New York: Shine Classics, 2014.

DiMascio, A., R. I. Shader and J. Harmatz. "Psychotropic Drugs and Induced Hostility." *Psychosomatics* 10(3)(May-June 1969):47-50. Accessed April 16, 2018. Quoted by Colin Downes-Grainger. "Medical Research on Benzodiazepine Injury." June 16, 2009. Accessed April 16, 2018. https://pdfs.semanticscholar.org/9227/c680079b542e3a7e650172bfc0bfbfb40f7b.pdf.

"Direct Tapers." BenzoBuddies. Accessed March 2, 2017. http://www.benzobuddies.org/benzodiazepine-withdrawal-methods/direct-taper/.

Downes-Grainger, Colin. "Medical Research on Benzodiazepine Injury." June 16, 2009. Accessed April 3, 2017. https://pdfs.semanticscholar.org/9227/c680079b542e3a7e650172bfc0bfbfb40f7b.pdf.

Downing, Nicholas S., Nilay D. Shah, Jenerius A. Aminawung, Alison M. Pease, Jean-David Zeitoun, Harlan M. Krumholz and Joseph S. Ross. "Postmarket Safety Events Among Novel Therapeutics Approved by the US Food and Drug Administration Between 2001 and 2010." *JAMA* 317(18)(May 9, 2017):1854-63. Accessed June 14, 2017. doi:10.1001/jama.2017.5150.

Drake. *Two Birds, One Stone*. Cash Money Records, 2016. https://genius.com/Drake-two-birds-one-stone-lyrics.

Duran Duran. *Lady Xanax*. Hollywood Records, 2000. https://www.azlyrics.com/lyrics/duranduran/ladyxanax.html.

The Escape Club. *Wild, Wild West*. WEA, 1988. https://genius.com/The-escape-club-wild-wild-west-lyrics.

Face the Facts. "Prescribed Addiction." BBC Radio 4. July 27, 2011. Last aired July 31, 2011. Produced by Kathryn Takatsuki. https://www.bbc.co.uk/programmes/b012wxxw.

Ferris Bueller's Day Off, DVD. Directed by John Hughes. Los Angeles: Paramount Pictures, 1986.

Fight Club. DVD. Directed by David Fincher. Los Angeles: Twentieth Century Fox, 1999.

Finding Nemo. DVD. Directed by Andrew Stanton and Lee Unkrich. Performed by Ellen DeGeneres. Screenplay by Andrew Stanton, Bob Peterson, and David Reynolds. 2003. Buena Vista Pictures, 2003.

Frances, Allen. "Yes, Benzos Are Bad for You." *Pro Talk: A Rehabs.com Community,* June 10, 2016. Accessed October 13, 2016. https://www.rehabs.com/pro-talk-articles/yes-benzos-are-bad-for-you/.

Fringe. "Unearthed." Directed by Frederick E. O. Toye. Written by David H. Goodman and Andrew Kreisberg. Warner Bros. Television, January 11, 2010.

"Generic Benzodiazepines and Brand Equivalents." *BenzoBuddies.* Accessed March 1, 2017. http://www.benzobuddies.org/benzodiazepine-information/benzo-list/.

Gibran, Kahlil. *The Prophet.* New York: Alfred A. Knopf, 1923.

Gorenstein, C., M. A. Bernik and S. Pompéia. "Differential Acute Psychomotor and Cognitive Effects of Diazepam on Long-Term Benzodiazepine Users." *International Clinical Psychopharmacology* 9(3)(1994):145-53. Accessed March 6, 2017. doi:10.1097/00004850-199409000-00002.

Gould, R. L., M. C. Coulson, N. Patel, E. Highton-Williamson and R. J. Howard. "Interventions for Reducing Benzodiazepine Use in Older People: Meta-Analysis of Randomised Controlled Trials." *British Journal of Psychiatry* 205(4)(2014):330. Accessed December 20, 2016. doi:10.1192/bjp.bp.113.126003.

Government of South Australia: Drug and Alcohol Services. "Benzodiazepine Equivalents." *SA Health.* DASSA:00107. August 2014. Accessed July 11, 2018. https://www.sahealth.sa.gov.au/wps/wcm/connect/83838b80407711959274ba22 2b2948cf/Benzodiazepine+equivalents-DASSA-August2014.pdf.

Halsey. *Colours.* Astralwerks, 2016. https://genius.com/Halsey-colors-lyrics.

Hammerschlag, Anke R, Sven Stringer, Christiaan A de Leeuw, Suzanne Sniekers, Erdogan Taskesen, Kyoko Watanabe, Tessa F Blanken, et al. "Genome-Wide Association Analysis of Insomnia Complaints Identifies Risk Genes and Genetic Overlap with Psychiatric and Metabolic Traits." Abstract. *Nature Genetics* 49 (2017): 1584-1592. doi:10.1038/ng.3888.

Helliwell, J., R. Layard and J. Sachs. *World Happiness Report 2017.* New York: Sustainable Development Solutions Network, 2017. http://worldhappiness.report/#happiness2017.

Higgitt, A., P. Fonagy, B. Toone and P. Shine. "The Prolonged Benzodiazepine Withdrawal Syndrome: Anxiety or Hysteria?" Abstract. *Acta Psychiatrica Scandinavica* 82(2)(August 1990):165-8. Accessed December 21, 2016. doi:10.1111/j.1600-0447.1990.tb01375.x.

Higgitt, A., M. H. Lader, P. Fonagy. "Clinical Management of Benzodiazepine Dependence." *British Medical Journal* 291(6497)(September 14, 1985):688-90. Accessed April 17, 2018. https://www.ncbi.nlm.nih.gov/pmc/articles/PMC1416639/.

Hirshkowitz, M. "The National Sleep Foundation's Sleep Time Duration Recommendations: Methodology and Results Summary." *Sleep Health* (2015). doi: 10.1016/j.sleh.2014.12.010.

Honoré, Carl. *In Praise of Slowness: Challenging the Cult of Speed.* New York: HarperOne, 2004.

The Hours. Directed by Stephen Daldry. Los Angeles: Paramount Pictures, 2002.

Huxley, Aldous. *Brave New World.* New York: Harper & Brothers, 1932. Print.

IMS Health. *Vector One: National (VONA) and Total Patient Tracker (TPT) Database* (2013). Extracted April 2014. Quoted in CCHR International. "Total Number of People Taking Psychiatric Drugs in the United States." Accessed April 3, 2018. https://www.cchrint.org/psychiatric-drugs/people-taking-psychiatric-drugs/.

In Pills We Trust. Discovery Channel. December 4-18, 2001. Quoted in "Professor Malcolm H Lader Quotations." *BenzoBuddies.* Accessed March 1, 2017. https://www.benzo.org.uk/lader2.htm.

Javed, Afzal. "Misuse of Benzodiazepine." *Journal of Pakistan Medical Association* 45(11)(November 1995):289-90. Accessed April 15, 2018. http://www.jpma.org.pk/full_article_text.php?article_id=4671.

Jay-Z and Alicia Keys. *Empire State of Mind.* Roc Nation, Atlantic, 2009. https://genius.com/Jay-z-empire-state-of-mind-lyrics.

Joughin, N., P. Tata, M. Collins, C. Hooper and J. Falkowski. "In-Patient Withdrawal from Long-Term Benzodiazepine Use." *British Journal of Addiction* 86(4)(April 1991):449-55. Accessed March 6, 2017. doi:10.1111/j.1360-0443.1991.tb03422.x.

Kierkegaard, Søren. *The Concept of Anxiety: A Simple Psychologically Orienting Deliberation on the Dogmatic Issue of Hereditary Sin.* Princeton, NJ: Princeton University Press, 1980.

Kim, Paul M. and Sujin Lee Weinstein. "Johns Hopkins Psychiatry Guide: Benzodiazepines." *Johns Hopkins Medicine.* Last updated May 8, 2015. Accessed April 9, 2018. https://www.hopkinsguides.com/hopkins/view/Johns_Hopkins_Psychiatry_Guide/787140/all/Benzodiazepines.

King, M.B. "Is There Still a Role for Benzodiazepines in General Practice?" *British Journal of General Practice* 42 (358): 202–5. Accessed March 6, 2017. PMC 1372025. https://www.ncbi.nlm.nih.gov/pmc/articles/PMC1372025/pdf/brjgenprac00056-0028.pdf.

Kottke, Leo. *Big Mob on the Hill.* Private Music, 1991. https://genius.com/Leo-kottke-big-mob-on-the-hill-lyrics.

Kripke, D. F., R.D. Langer and L.E. Kline. "Hypnotics' Association with Mortality or Cancer: A Matched Cohort Study." *BMJ Open* 2(e000850)(2012). Accessed June 21, 2017. doi:10.1136/bmjopen-2012-000850.

Lader, M. H. And S. V. Morton. "Benzodiazepine Problems." British Journal of Addiction 86(7)(July 1991):823-8. Accessed April 18, 2018. doi:10.1111/j.1360-0443.1991.tb01831.x.

Lader, M.H. and S.V. Morton. "A Pilot Study of the Effects of Flumazenil on Symptoms Persisting After Benzodiazepine Withdrawal." *Journal of Psychopharmacology* 6(3)(January 1992):357-63. Accessed March 6, 2017. doi:10.1177/026988119200600303.

Lader, Malcolm. "Anxiety or Depression During Withdrawal of Hypnotic Treatments." *Journal of Psychosomatic Research* 38(1)(1994):113-23. Accessed March 15, 2018. doi:10.1016/0022-3999(94)90142-2.

———. "Benzos and Memory Loss: More than Just 'Old Age.'" Reprint. *Prescriber* (February 1992). Accessed April 20, 2017. https://benzo.org.uk/amisc/ladermloss.pdf.

————. "History of Benzodiazepine Dependence." *Journal of Substance Abuse Treatment* 8 (1991):53-59. Accessed March 1, 2017. doi:10.1016/0740-5472(91)90027-8.

————. "Limitations on the Use of Benzodiazepines in Anxiety and Insomnia: Are They Justified?" *European Neuropsychopharmacology* 9(6)(December 1999):S399-405. PMID:10622686. https://www.ncbi.nlm.nih.gov/pubmed/?term=european+neuropsychopharmacology+1999+lader.

Lane, Christopher. "Brain Damage from Benzodiazepines: The Troubling Facts, Risks, and History of Minor Tranquilizers." *Psychology Today.* November 18, 2000. Accessed October 10, 2016. https://www.psychologytoday.com/us/blog/side-effects/201011/brain-damage-benzodiazepines-the-troubling-facts-risks-and-history-minor.

The Late Show Starring Stephen Colbert. Season 2, Episode 108. Starring Stephen Colbert. Written by Michael Pielocik. CBS, March 6, 2017.

Laufer, Offir, David Israeli and Rony Paz. "Behavioral and Neural Mechanisms of Overgeneralization in Anxiety." *Current Biology* 26 (March 21, 2016): 713-22, Accessed March 7, 2017. http://www.cell.com/current-biology/pdf/S0960-9822(16)00073-7.pdf.

Leclerq, Sophie, Paul Forsythe and John Bienenstock. "Prosttraumatic Stress Disorder: Does the Gut Microbiome Hold the Key?" *The Canadian Journal of Psychiatry: In Review Series* 61(4): 204-13, Accessed March 7, 2017. http://journals.sagepub.com/doi/pdf/10.1177/0706743716635535.

Lenhart, Amanda. "Teens, Social Media & Technology Overview 2015." *Pew Research Center Information & Technology* (April 9, 2015). Accessed April 6, 2018. http://www.pewinternet.org/2015/04/09/teens-social-media-technology-2015/.

Liebrenz, Michael, Marie-Therese Gehring, Anna Buadze and Carlo Caflisch. "High-Dose Benzodiazepine Dependence: A Qualitative Study of Patients' Perception on Cessation and Withdrawal." *BMC Psychiatry* 15(2015):116. Accessed April 11, 2018. doi:10.1186/s12888-015-0493-y.

Lil Peep. *Praying to the Sky.* 2015. https://genius.com/Lil-peep-praying-to-the-sky-lyrics.

Lil Wayne. *I Feel Like Dying.* No on Label (Lil Wayne), 2007. https://genius.com/Lil-wayne-i-feel-like-dying-lyrics.

Lil Wyte. *Oxy Cotton.* Hypnotize Minds, 2003. https://genius.com/Lil-wyte-oxy-cotton-lyrics.

Lin, Liu yi, Jaime E. Sidani, Ariel Shensa, Ana Radovic, Elizabeth Miller, Jason B. Colditz, Beth L. Hoffman, Leila M. Giles and Brian A. Primack "Association Between Social Media Use and Depression Among U.S. Young Adults." *Depression and Anxiety* (January 19, 2016). Accessed January 12, 2017. doi:10.1002/da.22466.

Lindskog, Anna-Lena. "Pharmaceutical Residue in Water Result in Bold and Voracious Perch." *Umea University: Faculty and Science Technology: About the Faculty: News.* February 14, 2013. Accessed March 6, 2017. http://www.teknat.umu.se/english/about-the-faculty/news/newsdetailpage//pharmaceutical-residue-in-water-result-in-bold-and-voracious-perch.cid208337#.

Longo, Lance P. and Brian Johnson. "Addiction: Part I. Benzodiazepines — Side Effects, Abuse Risk and Alternatives." *American Family Physician* 61(7)(April 1, 2000):2121-28. Accessed March 6, 2017. https://www.aafp.org/afp/2000/0401/p2121.html.

Maletzky, B. M. and J. Klotter. "Addiction to Diazepam." *International Journal of the Addictions* 11(1)(1976):95-115. Accessed April 17, 2018. https://www.ncbi.nlm.nih.gov/pubmed/1254372.

Marconi Union. "Weightless (Official Video)." Music video, 2014. Accessed April 13, 2018. https://www.youtube.com/watch?v=UfcAVejslrU.

Manson, Mark. *The Subtle Art of Not Giving a F*ck.* New York: HarperOne, 2016.

Maust, Donovan T., Helen C. Kales, Ilse R. Wiechers, Frederic C. Blow, Mark Olfson. "No End in Sight: Benzodiazepine Use in Older Adults in the United States." *Journal of the American Geriatrics Society* 64(12)(December 2016):2546-53. Accessed February 17, 2017. doi:10.1111/jgs.14379.

Maust, Donovan T., Lauren B. Gerlach, Anastasia Gibson, Helen C. Kales, Frederic C. Blow and Mark Olfson. "Trends in Central Nervous System — Active Polypharmacy Among Older Adults Seen in Outpatient Care in the United States." *JAMA Internal Medicine* 177(4)(April 2017):583-85. Accessed February 16, 2017. doi:10.1001/jamainternmed.2016.9225.

Mayer, John. *Heartbreak Warfare.* Columbia, 2010. https://genius.com/John-mayer-heartbreak-warfare-lyrics.

McCarthy, Justin. "More Americans Say Crime Is Rising in U.S." *Gallup.* October 22, 2015. Accessed April 12, 2018. http://news.gallup.com/poll/186308/americans-say-crime-rising.aspx.

Medical Council of Hong Kong (MCHK). *Guidelines on the Proper Prescription and Dispensing of Dangerous Drugs by Registered Medical Practitioners* (1996). Promulgated in April 1996.

Milton, John. *Paradise Lost.*

Morgan, Charles A., Sheila Wang, Ann Rasmusson, Gary Hazlett, George Anderson and Dennis Charney. "Relationship Among Plasma Cortisol, Catecholamine, Neuropeptide Y, and Human Performance During Exposure to Uncontrollable Stress." Abstract. *Psychosomatic Medicine* Vol. 63 Issue 3 (May-June 2001). 412-22. Accessed July 17, 2017. doi:10.1001/jamainternmed.2016.9225. https://journals.lww.com/psychosomaticmedicine/Abstract/2001/05000/Relations hip_Among_Plasma_Cortisol,.10.aspx.

Morrissey. *Something is Squeezing My Skull.* Polydor, 2009. https://genius.com/Morrissey-something-is-squeezing-my-skull-lyrics.

National Institute on Drug Abuse (NIDA). "Definition of Tolerance." *The Neurobiology of Drug Addiction.* Updated January 2007. Accessed August 6, 2017. https://www.drugabuse.gov/publications/teaching-packets/neurobiology-drug-addiction/section-iii-action-heroin-morphine/6-definition-tolerance.

National Institute on Drug Abuse (NIDA). "Is There a Difference Between Physical Dependence and Addiction?" *Principles of Drug Addiction Treatment: A Research-Based Guide (Third Edition).* Updated January 2018. Accessed April 8, 2018. https://www.drugabuse.gov/publications/principles-drug-addiction-treatment-research-based-guide-third-edition/frequently-asked-questions/there-difference-between-physical-dependence.

National Institute on Drug Abuse (NIDA). "Well-Known Mechanism Underlies Benzodiazepines' Addictive Properties." *NIDA Notes*, April 19, 2012. Accessed August 10, 2017. https://www.drugabuse.gov/news-events/nida-notes/2012/04/well-known-mechanism-underlies-benzodiazepines-addictive-properties.

New South Wales Government (NSW). "Benzodiazepines." *Health Fact Sheets*. Last updated July 11, 2013. Accessed March 6, 2017. http://www.health.nsw.gov.au/mentalhealth/Factsheets/Pages/benzodiazepines.aspx.

New York City Department of Health and Mental Hygiene (NYC DOHMH). *City Health Information: Judicious Prescribing of Benzodiazepines* 35(2)(2016). https://docs.wixstatic.com/ugd/990dad_167113513c9445f8bc77a77370ce649f.pdf.

OK Go. *A Million Ways.* Capitol Records, 2005. https://genius.com/Ok-go-a-million-ways-lyrics.

Olfson, M., M. King and M. Schoenbaum. "Benzodiazepine Use in the United States." *JAMA Psychiatry* 72(2)(February 2015):136-42. Accessed March 7, 2017. doi:10.1001/jamapsychiatry.2014.1763.

Oster, G., D. M. Huse, S. F. Adams, J. Imbimbo and M. W. Russell. "Benzodiazepine Tranquilizers and the Risk of Accidental Injury." *American Journal of Public Health* 80(12)(Dec 1990):1467-70. Accessed April 17, 2018. doi:10.2105/AJPH.80.12.1467. https://ajph.aphapublications.org/doi/pdf/10.2105/AJPH.80.12.1467.

"An Overview of Sleep Disorders." *Healthy Sleep: Division of Sleep Medicine at Harvard Medical School.* Last Updated December 18, 2007. Accessed March 7, 2017. http://healthysleep.med.harvard.edu/healthy/getting/treatment/an-overview-of-sleep-disorders.

Owens, M.J., M.A. Vargas and C.B. Nemeroff. "The Effects of Alprazolam on Corticotropin-Releasing Factor Neurons in the Rat Brain: Implications for a Role for CRF in the Pathogenesis of Anxiety Disorders." *Journal of Psychiatric Research* 27(1)(1993):209-20. Accessed March 6, 2017. PMID:8145178. https://www.ncbi.nlm.nih.gov/pubmed/?term=8145178.

Pariente, Antoine, Sophie Billioti de Gage, Nicholas Moore and Bernard Bégaud. "The Benzodiazepine–Dementia Disorders Link: Current State of Knowledge." *CNS Drugs* 30(1)(January 2016):1-7. Accessed December 12, 2016. doi:10.1007/s40263-015-0305-4.

Park, Bum Jin, Yuko Tsunetsugu, Tamami Kasetani, Takahide Kagawa and Yoshifumi Miyazaki. "The Physiological Effects of Shinrin-Yoku (Taking in the Forest Atmosphere or Forest Bathing): Evidence from Field Experiments in 24 Forests Across Japan." *Environmental Health and Preventive Medicine* 15(1)(January 2010):18-26. doi:10.1007/s12199-009-0086-9.

Pea, Roy, Clifford Nass, Lyn Meheula, Marcus Rance, Aman Kumar, Holden Bamford, Matthew Nass, Aneesh Simha, Benjamin Stillerman, Steven Yang and Michael Zhou, "Media Use, Face-to-Face Communication, Media Multitasking, and Social Well-Being Among 8- to 12-Year-Old Girls." Developmental Psychology 48(2) (2012): 327-36. Accessed February 20, 2017. doi:10.1037/a0027030.

Pétursson, H. And M. H. Lader. "Withdrawal from long-term benzodiazepine treatment." *British Medical Journal: Clinical Research Edition* 283(6292)(September 5, 1981:643-45. Accessed March 1, 2017. PMID:6114776. https://www.ncbi.nlm.nih.gov/pmc/articles/PMC1506756/pdf/bmjcred00675-0021.pdf.

Pétursson, Hafdan. "The Benzodiazepine Withdrawal Syndrome." *Addiction* 89(11)(November 1994):1455-59. Accessed March 6, 2017. PMID:7841856. https://www.ncbi.nlm.nih.gov/pubmed/7841856.

Pew Research Center Internet & Technology. "Social Media Fact Sheet." February 5, 2018. Accessed April 6, 2018. http://www.pewinternet.org/fact-sheet/social-media/.

Pill Friends. *Klonopin.* Pill Friends, 2014. https://genius.com/Pill-friends-klonopin-lyrics.

Pink Floyd. *Comfortably Numb.* New York: Columbia, 1979. https://www.discogs.com/Pink-Floyd-The-Wall/master/11329.

"Professor Malcolm H Lader: Quotations & CV." BenzoBuddies. Accessed March 1, 2017. https://www.benzo.org.uk/lader2.htm.

"Protracted Withdrawal Syndrome (PWS)." W-BAD. Accessed April 15, 2018. http://w-bad.org/protractedwithdrawalsyndrome/.

"PubChem Open Chemistry Database." NIH: U.S. National Library of Medicine: National Center for Biotechnology Information. (Access dates vary depending on drug being researched). https://pubchem.ncbi.nlm.nih.gov/.

Queens of the Stone Age. *Feel Good Hit of the Summer.* Interscope Records, 2000. https://genius.com/Queens-of-the-stone-age-feel-good-hit-of-the-summer-lyrics.

Ramster, D., A. J. Barber, A. Deb, K. Free, M. W. P. Carney and P. F. Ellis. "A Policy on Benzodiazepines." *The Lancet* 330(8572)(December 12, 1987):1406. Accessed April 17, 2018. doi:10.1016/S0140-6736(87)91304-3.

Rickels, K., W.G. Case, R.W. Downing and A. Winokur. "Long-Term Diazepam Therapy and Clinical Outcome."Abstract. *JAMA* 250(6)(August 12, 1983):767-71. Accessed March 1, 2017. PMID:6348314. https://www.ncbi.nlm.nih.gov/pubmed/6348314.

Reed, Lou. *Walk on the Wild Side.* RCA Victor, 1972. https://www.lyrics.com/lyric/4374579/Lou+Reed/Walk+on+the+Wild+Side.

Rolling Stones. *Mother's Little Helper.* London: London Records, 1966. https://www.discogs.com/The-Rolling-Stones-Mothers-Little-Helper-Lady-Jane/release/4528169.

Roser, Max and Esteban Ortiz-Ospina. "Global Extreme Poverty." *Our World in Data* (Online Resource). 2018. Accessed April 12, 2018. https://ourworldindata.org/extreme-poverty.

———. "Global Rise of Education." *Our World in Data* (Online Resource). 2017. Accessed April 12, 2018. https://ourworldindata.org/global-rise-of-education.

———. "Homicides." *Our World in Data* (Online Resource). 2018. Accessed April 12, 2018. https://ourworldindata.org/homicides.

Saarelainen, Laura, Anna-Maija Tolppanen, Marjaana Koponen, Antti Tanskanen, Jari Tiihonen, Sripa Hartikainen and Heidi Taipale. "Risk of Death Associated with New Benzodiazepine Use Among Persons with Alzheimer's Disease — a Matched Cohort Study." *International Journal of Geriatric Psychiatry* (November 15, 2017). Accessed April 8, 2018. doi:10.1002/gps.4821.

Scenic Train Ride from Bergen to Oslo (Norway). 1slowtv. Published August 30, 2014. Accessed November 23, 2016. https://www.youtube.com/watch?v=xisVS_DKpJg.

Shahly, Victoria, Patricia A. Berglund and Catherine Coulouvrat. "The Associations of Insomnia with Costly Workplace Accidents and Errors: Results from the America Insomnia Survey." *JAMA Psychiatry* 69(10) (October 2012):1054-1063. doi:10.1001/archgenpsychiatry.2011.2188.

Shantideva. *Guide to the Bodhisattva's Way of Life: A Buddhist Poem for Today.* New York: Tharpa Publications, 2002.

Silver Linings Playbook. Directed by David O. Russell. New York: The Weinstein Company, 2012.

The Simpsons. "Crook and Ladder." Directed by Lance Kramer. Written by Bill Odenkirk. 20th Century Fox Television, May 6, 2007.

Smith, Emily Esfahani. "There's More to Life Than Being Happy." *TED Talk.* April 2017. Accessed April 13, 2018. https://www.ted.com/talks/emily_esfahani_smith_there_s_more_to_life_than_being_happy.

Smith, R. J. "Study Finds Sleeping Pills Overprescribed." *Science* 204(4390)(April 20, 1979):287-8. Accessed April 17, 2018. doi:10.1126/science.219479.

Spence, D. Warren, Leonid Kayumov, Adam Chen, Alan Lowe, Umesh Jain, Martin A. Katzman, Jianhua Shen, Boris Perelman, and Colin M. Shapiro. "Acupuncture Increases Nocturnal Melatonin Secretion and Reduces Insomnia and Anxiety: A Preliminary Report." *The Journal of Neuropsychiatry and Clinical Neurosciences.* Special Article (February 1, 2004). Accessed July 11, 2018. https://neuro.psychiatryonline.org/doi/full/10.1176/jnp.16.1.19.

Starting Over. DVD. Directed by Alan J. Pakula. Los Angeles: Paramount Pictures, 1979.

Stossel, Scott. *My Age of Anxiety: Fear, Hope, Dread, and the Search for Peace of Mind.* New York: Vintage Books, 2013.

Tan, Kelly R., Matthew Brown, Gwenaël Labouèbe, Cédric Yvon, Cyril Creton, Jean-Marc Fritschy, Uwe Rudolph and Christian Lüscher. "Neural Bases for Addictive Properties of Benzodiazepines." Abstract. *Nature* 463: 769-74 (February 11, 2010). Accessed August 10, 2017. doi:10.1038/nature08758.

Tata, P.R., J. Rollings, M. Collins, A. Pickering and R. R. Jacobson. "Lack of Cognitive Recovery Following Withdrawal from Long-Term Benzodiazepine Use." *Psychological Medicine* 24(1)(February 1994):203-13. Accessed April 15, 2018. doi:10.1017/S0033291700026969.

The Tranquillisers Trap. BBC-1. May 1, 2013. Transcribed from a transcription unit recording, not original script. Reported by Shelley Jofre. Produced by Murdoch Rodgers. Assistant Producers Tom Anstiss and Rob Cole. Accessed March 4, 2017. http://news.bbc.co.uk/hi/english/static/audio_video/programmes/panorama/transcripts/transcript_13_05_01.txt.

Trickett, Shirley. "Withdrawal from Benzodiazepines." *Journal of the Royal College of General Practitioners* 33(254)(September 1983):608. Accessed April 17, 2018. https://www.ncbi.nlm.nih.gov/pmc/articles/PMC1973010/.

U.K. Department of Health (DH). *Benzodiazepines Warning: A Communication to All Doctors from the Chief Medical Officer: CMO's Update* 37(January 2004).

U.K. National Health Service (NHS). "Guidance for Prescribing and Withdrawal of Benzodiazepines & Hypnotics in General Practice." *NHS Grampian*. October 2006. Reviewed October 2008. https://www.benzo.org.uk/amisc/bzgrampian.pdf.

U.K. National Institute for Health and Care Excellence (NICE). *NICE Guidance: Anxiety Disorders: Quality Statement 3: Pharmacological Treatment* (QS53)(February 2014). Accessed April 10, 2018. https://www.nice.org.uk/guidance/qs53/chapter/quality-statement-3-pharmacological-treatment.

U.S. Centers for Disease Control and Prevention (CDC). "Deaths: Final Data for 2015." *National Vital Statistics Reports* 66(6)(November 27, 2017). https://www.cdc.gov/nchs/data/nvsr/nvsr66/nvsr66_06.pdf.

U.S. Centers for Disease Control and Prevention (CDC). "Drugs Most Frequently Involved in Drug Overdose Deaths: United States, 2010–2014." *National Vital Statistics Reports* 65(10)(December 20, 2016). https://www.cdc.gov/nchs/data/nvsr/nvsr65/nvsr65_10.pdf.

U.S. Centers for Disease Control and Prevention (CDC). "Leading Causes of Death in Males (2014)" *Health Equity* (Last Updated January 26, 2017). Accessed April 6, 2018. https://www.cdc.gov/healthequity/lcod/men/2014/index.htm.

U.S. Department of Commerce: International Trade Administration (ITA). *2016 Top Markets Report Pharmaceuticals: Overview and Key Findings*. Accessed April 13, 2017. https://www.trade.gov/topmarkets/pdf/Pharmaceuticals_Executive_Summary.pdf.

U.S. Department of Veteran's Affairs (VA/DoD). *PTSD: National Center for PTSD: Use of Benzodiazepines for PTSD in Veterans Affairs*. Accessed June 21, 2017. https://www.ptsd.va.gov/professional/treatment/overview/benzo-ptsd-va.asp.

U.S. Drug Enforcement Administration (DEA). *Drug Info: Drug Scheduling*. Accessed March 2, 2018. https://www.dea.gov/druginfo/ds.shtml.

U.S. Drug Enforcement Administration (DEA). *Office of Diversion Control; Drug & Chemical Evaluation Section: Benzodiazepines* (January 2013). Accessed March 6, 2017. https://www.deadiversion.usdoj.gov/drug_chem_info/benzo.pdf.

U.S. Food & Drug Administration (FDA). "FDA Drug Safety Communication: FDA Updates Warnings for Oral and Injectable Fluoroquinolone Antibiotics Due to Disabling Side Effects." *Drug Safety: Safety Announcement* (September 26, 2016). Last updated March 8, 2018. Accessed April 10, 2018. https://www.fda.gov/Drugs/DrugSafety/ucm511530.htm.

U.S. Food & Drug Administration (FDA). "FDA Requires Strong Warnings for Opioid Analgesics, Prescription Opioid Cough Products, and Benzodiazepine Labeling Related to Serious Risks and Death from Combined Use." *FDA News Release* (August 31, 2016). Last Updated August 31, 2016. Accessed September 21, 2017. https://www.fda.gov/NewsEvents/Newsroom/PressAnnouncements/ucm518697.htm.

Ventola, C. Lee. "Direct-to-Consumer Pharmaceutical Advertising: Therapeutic or Toxic?" *Pharmacy and Therapeutics* 36(10)(October 2011):669-74, 681-84. Accessed August 29, 2017. https://www.ncbi.nlm.nih.gov/pmc/articles/PMC3278148/.

Vertosick Jr., Frank. *When the Air Hits Your Brain: Tales from Neurosurgery*. New York: W. W. Norton & Company, 1996.

Weng, Chuan-Bo, Ruo-Bing Qian, Zian-Ming Fu, Bin Lin, Xiao-Peng Han, Chao-Shi Niu and Ye-Han Wang. "Gray Matter and White Matter Abnormalities in Online Game Addiction." Abstract. *European Journal of Radiology* 82(8) (Aug 2013): 1308-12. Accessed April 6, 2018. doi: 10.1016/j.ejrad.2013.01.031.

World Health Organization (WHO). *Cannabidiol (CBD): Pre-Preview Report: Expert Committed on Drug Dependence (ECDD)* 39th Meeting (Geneva, November 6-10, 2017). Accessed April 13, 2018. http://www.who.int/medicines/access/controlled-substances/5.2_CBD.pdf.

World Health Organization (WHO). *Depression and Other Common Mental Disorders: Global Health Estimates* 2017.2. License: CC BY-NC-SA 3.0 IGO. Accessed April 5, 2018. http://apps.who.int/iris/bitstream/handle/10665/254610/WHO-MSD-MER-2017.2-eng.pdf;jsessionid=6EE9A59935A104950FF3C57F106F0D65?sequence=1.

World Health Organization (WHO). *Mental Health in the Workplace: Information Sheet* (September 2017). Accessed April 5, 2018. http://www.who.int/mental_health/in_the_workplace/en/.

Comments? Feedback? Share Your Story?

We'd love to hear from you.

Please visit us at
www.BenzoFree.org/Feedback

Made in the USA
Columbia, SC
01 October 2023

23692805R00205